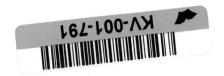

Postural Disorders and Musculoskeletal Dysfunction

DIAGNOSIS, PREVENTION AND TREATMENT

Dr. Gill Solberg Ph.D
Lecturer, Kibbutzim College of Education;
Lecturer, Zinman College of Physical Education and Sports
Sciences at The Wingate Institute, Israel.
Private practitioner www.solberg.co.il

Forewords by
Dr. Vardita Gur
Head, Posture Cultivation Department, and Director,
Center for Posture Treatment, Zinman College of Physical Education and Sport,
The Wingate Institute, Israel

and

Dr. Eli Adar
Director, Arthroscopic Orthopedic Department, and
Director, Clinic for Sport Injuries, Wolfson Medical Center, Holon, Israel

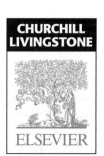

Edinburgh London New York Oxford Philadelphia St Louis Sydney Toronto 2008

CHURCHILL
LIVINGSTONE
ELSEVIER

An imprint of Elsevier Limited

© 2005, Dr. Gill Solberg
© 2008, Elsevier Limited. All rights reserved.

Originally published in Hebrew

The right of Dr. Gill Solberg to be identified as author of this work has been asserted by him in accordance with the Copyright, Designs and Patents Act 1988.

First edition 2005
Second edition 2008

ISBN: 978-0-443-10382-7

British Library Cataloguing in Publication Data
A catalogue record for this book is available from the British Library

Library of Congress Cataloging in Publication Data
A catalog record for this book is available from the Library of Congress

Note
Neither the Publisher nor the Author assumes any responsibility for any loss or injury and/or damage to persons or property arising out of or related to any use of the material contained in this book. It is the responsibility of the treating practitioner, relying on independent expertise and knowledge of the patient, to determine the best treatment and method of application for the patient.

The Publisher

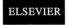 **ELSEVIER** your source for books, journals and multimedia in the health sciences
www.elsevierhealth.com

Working together to grow
libraries in developing countries

www.elsevier.com | www.bookaid.org | www.sabre.org

ELSEVIER   BOOK AID International   Sabre Foundation

The publisher's policy is to use paper manufactured from sustainable forests

Printed in China

Contents

Forewords

This book is the jewel in the crown of a consistent and soundly-based process of professional development. It is undoubtedly an expression of self-fulfillment by a professional whose path has been characterized by study, expanding knowledge and varied experience.

This is the first book of its type on posture. It is intended to raise public awareness about a subject that has been shunted to the sidelines and to a certain extent snubbed by orthopedics, physical therapy and physical education – the fields that are supposed to deal with it.

Orthopedists recognize the existence of posture, but except for cases requiring treatment entailing a brace or surgery, the attitude is one of general avoidance. This attitude derives from a view of postural problems as a matter of aesthetics or behavior, to which orthopedics has no commitment because they do not pose a danger to life or general functioning. Physical therapy treats posture with a modicum of respect but its daily routine encounters such a broad range of musculoskeletal problems that there is little time to deal with posture. On the other hand, physical education and its various subdivisions recognize, respect, and even like to deal with the subject, but too often without the theoretical basis necessary for constructing a responsible, controlled therapeutic system.

This book provides the thread that connects these three domains. It is written with respect for all those who engage in the field and it advocates an approach in which all three domains can unite and together contribute to creating a comprehensive therapeutic system. In each aspect of the issues discussed in the book, the author takes great care to use relevant professional language. Readers, regardless of their professional bent, can find chapters that are of direct benefit to them, and others that supplement and fill in missing knowledge. Although the author's specialization is the therapeutic movement approach to posture, he systemically and in good didactic fashion presents:

1. Basic concepts in the kinesiology and biomechanics of posture.
2. Concise orthopedic dimensions.
3. Theory-based principles of diagnosis and treatment.

These principles, with their shared theoretical basis, can be molded into a number of different work approaches, depending on each therapist's tendency and relevant considerations in each case.

The book neither confuses nor blurs the boundaries between familiar kinesiological and physiological principles and common treatment approaches. Moreover, the author makes no claim to having personally formulated the principles he presents. Throughout the book, the author remains true to his aim of increasing posture awareness by expanding related knowledge, without setting up posture as the be-all and end-all, and without trumpeting, as the final word, the treatment methods he presents.

The book does not enter into discussions of controversial issues and it does not expand on orthopedic matters because from the outset this was not the author's intention. At the same time, he opens a window onto a world in which questions abound, letting in needed air for refreshing readers' thinking processes about posture and about modes of application. He also invites the professional reader to supplement, add, subtract, and connect.

I am especially fond of Gill's motto, reflected in a quotation from Irvin Yalom: "The strong temptation to find certainty by adopting a given ideal school of thought or rigid system of treatment – is traitorous."

Well done!

Dr. Vardita Gur
Head, Posture Cultivation Department, and Director, Center for Posture Treatment, Zinman College of Physical Education and Sport, The Wingate Institute, Israel.

I read Dr. Solberg's book with great pleasure. One especially stimulating aspect of this book is the fact that it can be read both by professionals and lay people who wish to understand the approaches to treating children with postural disorders. What is especially important is the author's emphasis on the child's enjoyment during treatment as a tool to ensure continued participation and improvement.

Children with posture and motoric disabilities have their own independent personalities with desires and likes of their own. In treating them, we must not ignore these. We must preserve their personalities by revealing their abilities and by endowing them with the tools they need to improve these abilities.

The underlying aim is to help these children to integrate with their peers, and prepare them to enter society in the future. When children are aware of their functional limitations and as a result refrain from participating in society, it is important to inculcate in them the idea that "throwing the ball at the basket is more important than getting it through the hoop". Working on performance quality will come later when the children demand it, when they internalize the need to improve their performance.

Dr. Solberg's book provides the tools required for helping children to progress both affectively and motorically. The author repeatedly emphasizes that the exercises he presents are not an end in themselves, and that they are intended to help the individual child to progress. To know which exercises should be adapted for which patients, it is important for therapists to know and understand the children they work with, and to approach them as complete individual entities.

Dr. Eli Adar
Director, Arthroscopic Orthopedic Department, and Director, Clinic for Sport Injuries, Wolfson Medical Center, Holon, Israel.

Preface

The story of the frog that got cooked

Once upon a time there was a frog known for its ability to "adapt". It could live at the North Pole and it could live in the desert; it climbed trees and plumbed the depths of rivers, and wherever it went it adapted to whatever conditions prevailed. Its "adapt-ability" was so impressive that a special committee of animals in the forest convened to discuss the possibility of appointing the frog to the position of "World Adviser for Adaptive Affairs". But, before being awarded such a prestigious post, the frog had to pass a test. It was placed in a pool of shallow water that warmed by one degree every minute. What the frog had to do was to adapt to the water, and after it had attained the maximal rate of adaptation – it could jump out any time it wanted. So the frog adapted, and adapted, and adapted … until … it was cooked!

Relationships are the healers (Irvin Yalom)

The dilemma of when to jump out confronts the therapist constantly. The therapeutic process, in any field, requires professional deliberation as to which path to choose, but this is not enough. After the path has been chosen and the process has begun, the therapist may begin to feel comfortable, warm, and secure in the chosen path, even if, over time, the path is no longer suitable and needs to be altered – in other words, it's time to "jump out" and stop adapting.

The ability to live with uncertainty and to change therapeutic direction is a prerequisite for engaging in a therapeutic profession. Even though many professionals guide their patients systematically and with a sure hand towards a pre-established goal, a good therapist often has doubts, improvises, and seeks direction.

In his book *Love's Hangman* (1991), Irvin Yalom writes: "The strong temptation to find certainty by adopting a given ideal school of thought or rigid system of treatment – is traitorous. Such a belief may impede the spontaneous and uncertain encounter that is necessary for therapeutic success. This encounter, the heart of hearts of therapy, is a profound and caring encounter between two people."

A "100% guaranteed" method or exercise that brought about such impressive success with one patient may drop us onto a bed of humiliating failure with another patient. Therefore, one of the aims of this book is to set down a number of principles that encourage flexible thinking in the work of teachers or therapists treating individuals with postural disorders. This will hopefully help therapists to remain aware of and attuned to the complexity of the therapeutic process and to the constant changes occurring in them and in their patients, changes that therapists must adapt to without getting cooked …

Israel 2007   Gill Solberg

Acknowledgments

Many people helped me in writing this book. First, my thanks to my lovely daughters, Roni and Michal, who had to suffer through the hundreds of hours when all they could see of me was my back bent over the computer keyboard. Both of them succeeded in performing and modelling the exercises presented in this book with great wisdom and patience. To them go my heartfelt thanks; and to my wife, Orly, who at times believed in me more than I believed in myself.

To Dr. Vardita Gur, head of the Posture Cultivation Department at the Zinman College of Physical Education at The Wingate Institute, who read the book a number of times and who, with great professional insight bolstered by rich therapeutic experience, helped me to present the material in the proper light. To Dr. Efrat Heiman, head of the Physical Education and Movement Department at the Seminar Hakibbutzim Teachers College, who read the entire manuscript and offered her professional criticism. To Dr. Eli Adar of the Orthopedic Department of Wolfson Hospital, who allowed me to observe his skilled work during orthopedic examinations of children with special needs and to learn from his rich experience. Dr. Adar devoted many hours to reading the text and contributed to a balanced presentation of the subject from the medical viewpoint.

Thanks to Professor Chartris of the Clinical Kinesiology Department of Rhodes University, South Africa, for his professional guidance in the subjects dealing with posture examinations and ways of diagnosing scoliosis, and to Michael and to Garmise, the translator, who toiled successfully to translate the original text into English.

Special thanks to Noam and Ronen, of Studio Ze, for their patience and professionalism in the graphic editing of the book. During the many months of working with them, they did not compromise on a single detail and spared no effort to make each detail as perfect as possible. Thanks to Dave Helpman and Gershon Waldman for their professionalism, and the pleasant atmosphere they created during the long photographic sessions for the book.

And finally, to my mother, Rachel Solberg, who established the Yoga Teachers' Association in Israel and the first School for Integrative Yoga Teachers. Her rich experience as a teacher provided the basis for my professional development.

Introduction

This book grew out of a personal need to chart a comprehensive integrative approach to treating postural disorders. During my work as a diagnostician and therapist, I am constantly confronted with the challenge of understanding how the entire array of components connected to individuals' personality affects – and is affected by – their posture.

I have seen many professionals who try to treat a postural disorder by simplifying the issue and "isolating" it from the locomotor system, as if it were some kind of "static independent entity". The approach in this book is different. It sees posture as a dynamic, complex process that is influenced by and also influences the entire ensemble of domains that make up the human personality. This approach, of course, also impacts upon the development of the diagnostic and therapeutic means discussed in this work.

Most of the material presented in this book was collected and processed in the last few years. The ideas you will find here took shape in a number of places: at Rhodes University, South Africa, where I spent 2 years doing research; at the Center for Therapeutic Sport in Holon, Israel, where I served as a therapist and diagnostician; at the Zinman College of Physical Education at The Wingate Institute, where I lecture in the Posture Cultivation Department; and at the Kibbutzim College of Education, where I lecture in the Department of Physical Education for Populations with Special Needs. In this book, I sought to set down most of the basic information needed by teachers, instructors or therapists working with people with postural disorders. I tried to arrange the material in a way that facilitated an easy integration of the theoretical and the practical in therapy. The practical material is divided into a number of areas so that therapists/instructors can concentrate on one specific subject or another at any given time, according to their special needs of the moment. It is not my intention to equip teachers and therapists with a technical list of exercises that will form the only basis for their work. Rather, it is my desire to help therapists develop something themselves, by listening and attending to their patients' personality structure and changing needs.

By internalizing the material presented here and combining it with experience in the field, they will be able to generate a personal synthesis molded to and by their experience. The therapeutic process is not a sequence of exercises just as a wall is not a pile of bricks. In other words, just as a wall built only of bricks will topple, posture therapy based only on exercises will not yield results over time.

To build and stabilize their "therapeutic wall", therapists must make use of the "mortar" that amalgamates the bricks. Only the balanced combination and integration of mortar and bricks will ensure stability over time.

When working on posture, the purpose of physical exercise is to enable patients to stabilize themselves (by developing strength, muscle endurance, and normal ranges of motion). However, these are only the "bricks" that, in and of themselves, are insufficient. The course of therapy must emphasize other aspects – the "mortar", if you will – aspects that pertain to modifying postural habits and deficient movement patterns. Without proper attention to these aspects, patients will not alter the movement patterns ingrained in their nervous systems, and will persist in their deficient acquired manners of movement.

To this end, the book emphasizes an integrative approach to treating postural disorders, which encourages the use of other "tools" in addition to exercises. These "tools" are detailed throughout the book and can be presented graphically as follows:

Integrative treatment for improving movement and postural patterns					
Physical awareness and relaxation	Posture exercises and therapeutic exercise	Massages to release tension spots	Passive movement to improve ranges of motion	Hydrotherapy and therapeutic swimming	Guided touch and resistance exercises

Before a process of postural change can actually occur, individuals must be aware of their situation and, of course, have the desire to change it. Then, the first step is to teach them to be aware of their body and afterwards to use it properly. Treatment is intended to improve bodily function as a whole entity and not to cure the isolated symptom of a specific problem alone. Therefore, regular physical "exercises" serve only as partial means for attaining this goal.

I hope, through this book, to be of service to my fellow practitioners by presenting them with a helpful array of therapeutic ideas and principles.

CHAPTER 1

The integrative approach to posture

Movement and postural patterns are important components in a child's physical and emotional development. Movement is usually perceived as flowing and dynamic, while posture is seen as a static state characterized by lack of movement. But regarding posture as an independent factor unconnected to the overall functioning of the locomotor system is fundamentally wrong. The word "posture" means a position in which the whole body, or part of it, is held. A "multi-limbed" dynamic organism such as the human body cannot be defined as having only one posture. It takes on many positions, only rarely holding any one of them for very long.

The basic and most important function of the skeletal and muscular system is movement, and any static state in which the body finds itself is only part of this basic activity, since posture "follows" movement like a shadow. Expanding on this idea, Roaf (1978) defined posture as "a temporary position" assumed by the body in preparation for the next position. Therefore, static standing is not "real" posture, as we hold such a position so rarely.

To discuss the broad essence of the term "posture", we must address a number of the factors affecting it (Fig. 1.1).

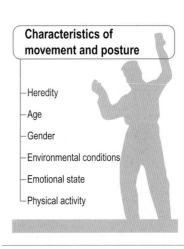

Characteristics of movement and posture

— Heredity

— Age

— Gender

— Environmental conditions

— Emotional state

— Physical activity

Figure 1.1 Factors affecting movement and postural patterns.

Kinesiological and other factors affecting human posture

Heredity

The genetic cargo people are born with affects their physical development and postural patterns. Details such as physique (ectomorphic, mesomorphic, endomorphic) and the length and weight of bones are givens at birth and together comprise a dominant factor in postural development.

Age

Postural patterns change during the life cycle, from the moment of birth, through all stages of development and into old age. Cogent examples of these changes can be seen mainly in:

Therapeutic cookbooks offering a fixed exercise recipe for each problem are written by people who do not allow facts to interfere with reality

- The gradual development of the structure of the foot arches
- The position of the lower extremity joints
- Changes in the angles pertaining to the anatomical structure of the femur (see the neck shaft angle, Fig. 5.7, and the torsion angle, Fig. 5.10 in Ch. 5)
- The position and stability of the pelvis
- Development of the spinal curves
- Stability of the shoulder girdle.

In this context, one should be aware of the changes occurring in patients during treatment and adapt it to changing needs. In other words, yesterday's exercise program is not necessarily appropriate for the patient today. This is reminiscent of Heraclites' famous dictum: "Everything flows." According to Heraclites, one cannot enter the same river twice. His pupils went so far as to state that no-one can ever enter the same flowing river even once. And from my viewpoint as a therapist, I would add that the river cannot flow over the same person twice because each moment it is flowing over a different person.

Gender

Several dissimilarities are evident between the posture of men and of women and are generally attributable to anatomical and physiological differences. These variations are especially visible in the following examples (Gould & Davies, 1985):

- A greater lumbar pelvic angle among women (which affects the position of the pelvis and the lumbar spinal column)
- Higher percentages of fat tissue in women (which has an overall effect on body structure and postural patterns).

Environmental conditions

Environmental conditions affect all areas in which human beings conduct their lives, among them:

- Work environment – the job one holds, the activities performed during the day, even prevailing dressing habits (a tailored suit, high heels or casual clothes?) have a cumulative effect on postural and movement patterns (Hales & Bernard, 1996).
- Social factors – including social norms affect posture such as the way people walk and dress, etc. Examples might be the "relaxed" posture favored by teenagers, the slouching walk affected by fashion models or the ramrod erectness of military officers.

Emotional state

Postural patterns are a visual clue to emotional state. From early developmental stages, movement patterns become so intertwined with emotional and cognitive impressions that the cumulative muscular stress in the body can be seen as a mirror of the body's expression. People experiencing emotional stress, anxiety, grief or lack of confidence, bear their bodies in a manner that externally reflects these feelings.

Where these interrelationships persist over long periods of time, the result may be habitual patterns. In other words, emotional processes may help to perpetuate fixated bodily patterns. In this book's integrative approach, effective movement therapy for postural disorders is based on physical exercise that addresses the psychomotor domain as well. As noted, in this approach the physical, the emotional, and the cognitive, constitute a multidimensional entity that finds its expression in postural patterns.

Physical activity

Adapted physical activity may contribute to normal development and to improving movement and postural patterns, but in cases where activities do not maintain body balance, the result may be functional limitations and impairment of optimal movement patterns.

The movement approach presented in this book is a synthesis of systems from both Eastern and Western philosophies and is based on widely accepted kinesiological and biomechanical principles.

Main aspects of normal posture

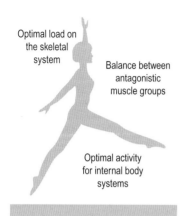

Figure 1.2 Main aspects of normal posture.

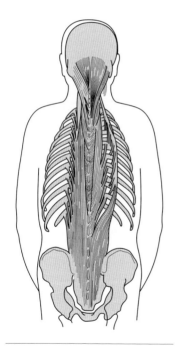

Figure 1.3 Antagonistic muscle groups in the back.

We have seen that the term posture, with its psychological, kinesiological, biomechanical, and physiological implications, represents a whole conglomeration of domains. This complexity has provoked much disagreement about the definition, diagnosis, and means of treating various disorders (Gur, 1998a). The professional literature on the subject is brimming with subjective "definitions" of normal posture ("good" posture, "bad" posture).

In this book, I do not use terms like "ideal", "good", or "bad" because they have no independent meaning, and definitions such as "good posture" or "bad posture" that are subjectively applied to different postures by different people are not sufficient. What might suit a 17-year-old with an ectomorphic physique is not necessarily suitable to a 12-year-old with an endomorphic somatotype. In other words, it is almost impossible to find a universal norm that reflects a posture that is "good" or "ideal" for all.

The approach offered here for treating postural disorders views each person as a unique individual, and tries to improve that person's physical state in relation to itself, without attempting to impose "accepted standards" subjectively determined by one researcher or another. Nevertheless, certain functional aspects taken together may be seen as basic "principles" for normal posture (Fig. 1.2).

Three of these principles are prerequisites for normal posture:

1. Optimal load on the skeletal system

   Despite its physical rigidity, bone tissue is dynamic in nature and responds to loads imposed on it. The study of bone growth indicates that bone grows in direct proportion to the load placed on it, within physiological limits.

   In postural disorders, there is an imbalance in the loads imposed on different areas. In these situations where loads exceed normal physiological limits consistently and over prolonged periods of time, structural changes occur in the skeletal bones. Damage of this type is usually irreversible (Norkin & Levangie, 1993).

2. Balance between antagonistic muscle groups

   Constant muscle tone facilitates balance and stability in body joints. In normal posture, antagonistic muscle groups work in different directions in order to stabilize the body and keep it in a state of balance. Upsetting this functional balance between opposing muscle groups may lead in time to the development of postural disorders (Kendall & McCreary, 1983) (Fig. 1.3).

3. Optimal activity for internal body systems

    Long-term postural disorders may also impair the normal functioning of internal body systems. This emphasizes the fact that maintenance of body health depends first and foremost upon proper functioning of internal systems and not necessarily on the functioning of the muscular system.

    Postural disorders, the primary symptoms of which are often detected in the skeletal system, create negative chain reactions over time that affect the functioning of other systems as well. The most vulnerable systems as a result of postural disorders are:

    - The respiratory system (mainly in states of kyphosis and scoliosis, because of pressure on the chest cavity)
    - The nervous system (which is affected mainly by pathologies connected to the functioning of the cervical, thoracic or lumbar vertebrae of the spine)
    - The digestive system (in situations entailing defective positioning of the pelvis and weakness of the abdominal and lower pelvic muscles)
    - The circulatory system (in disorders that interfere with normal blood flow as a result of malalignment of the various joints).

CHAPTER 2

Anatomical and kinesiological basis of posture

Anatomically, posture is dependent on the interaction of the skeletal, muscular and non-contractive connective tissue systems (including fascia, tendons and ligaments). Biomechanically, the complex stress structure of complementary forces created by these three systems also makes erect, balanced posture possible. For this reason, theoretical material about the anatomy, biomechanics and kinesiology of posture is included in this book.

Knowledge in these areas will enable therapists to work confidently and base their work on an understanding of the body's movement, while also reducing the likelihood of causing damage through improper exercises. Professionals engaging in movement therapy must be well versed in the

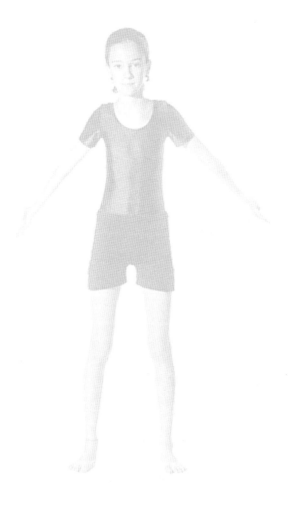

factors affecting the performance of each exercise – this is a prerequisite for proper, responsible treatment.

As with the therapeutic process, a sound knowledge of anatomy of the movement system cannot be learned only from books or by examining anatomical charts and models. Knowledge of anatomy is acquired through systematic work and extensive experience. Observing, listening, asking questions, and, of course, hands-on practice, are the main ways through which such knowledge can be internalized and then applied.

The study of anatomy can be divided into descriptive anatomy, which systematically describes the anatomical structure of the body in great detail, and topographic anatomy, which deals with the make-up of the body in terms of local relationships between organs situated in a given area. This chapter presents the applied aspects of both descriptive and topographic anatomy with special reference to the kinesiology of human posture (movement emphases that clarify functional connections between body joints). In addition, this chapter will also describe the function of the nervous system in maintaining posture.

This combination of an applied anatomy review with kinesiological emphases is intended to make it easier for readers to integrate posture-relevant material, so that they can further expand their knowledge and compare practice to theory.

Basic movement terms

Flexion

Extension

Adduction

Abduction

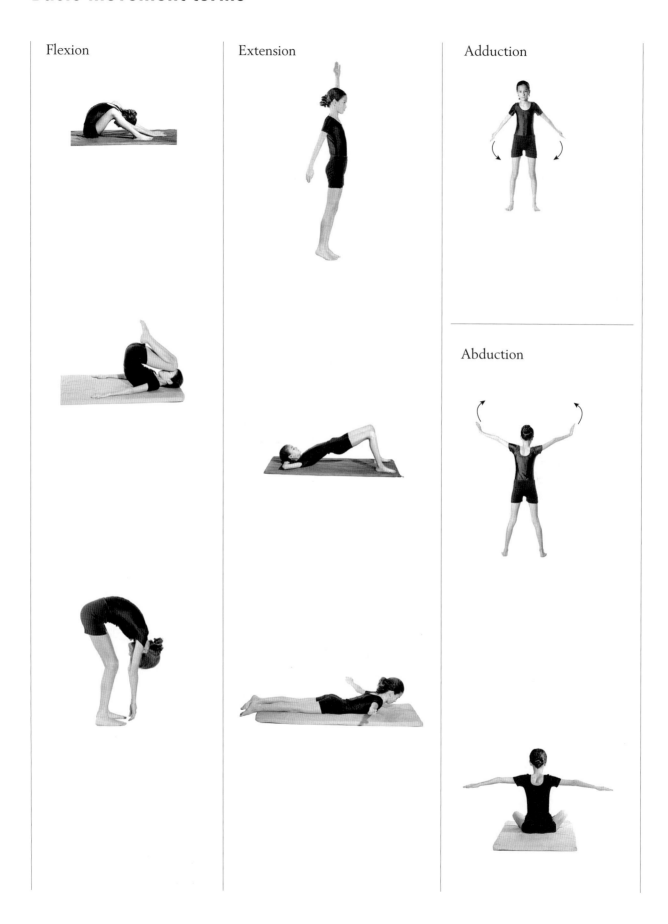

External/internal rotation

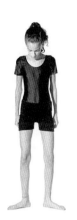

Dorsiflexion

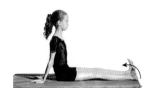

Eversion

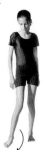

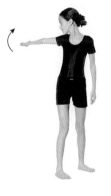

Plantar flexion

Inversion

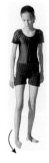

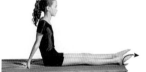

Protraction

Retraction

Elevation

Depression

Scapular adduction

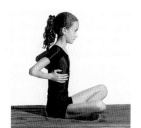

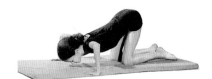

Scapular abduction

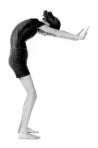

Anterior/posterior pelvic tilt (see Fig. 2.1)

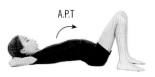

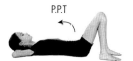

Movement refers to the ASIS – anterior superior iliac spine. Posterior pelvic tilt (PPT) entails a flattening of lumbar lordosis and bringing the hip joints forward. Anterior pelvic tilt (APT) involves an increase in lumbar lordosis (Fig. 2.1).

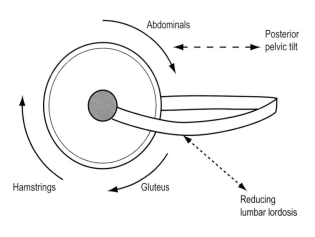

Figure 2.1 The mechanism of anterior and posterior pelvic tilt.

Movement planes in the human body

Body movements are performed in the following three planes:

1. Movements in the sagittal plane, e.g.
Flexion
Extension.

2. Movements in the coronal/frontal plane, e.g.
Abduction
Adduction
Lateral flexion.

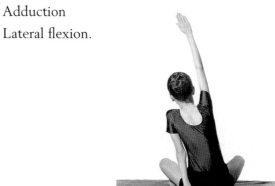

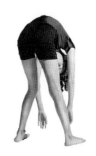

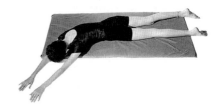

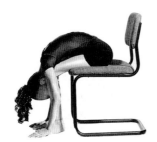

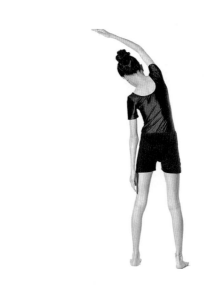

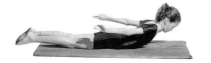

3. Movements in the horizontal plane, e.g.
External/Lateral rotation
Internal/Medial rotation
Spinal rotation.

4. Movement in all the planes, e.g.
Full revolutions of the shoulder joint
(Circumduction).

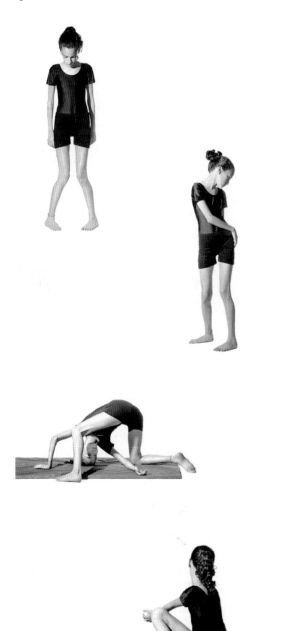

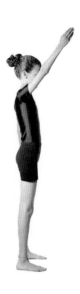

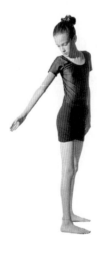

The muscular system: anatomical and kinesiological aspects of maintaining posture

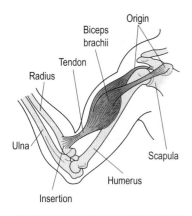

Figure 2.2 Origin and insertion of the biceps brachii muscle.

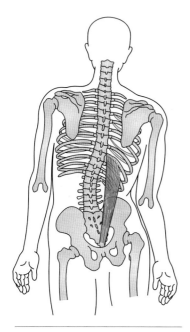

Figure 2.3 Example of imbalance between antagonistic muscles creating scoliosis in the spine (Nudelman & Reis, 1990). Additional causes of scoliosis are detailed in Chapter 4.

Normal movement functioning of the human body depends on a stable and balanced muscular system that supports the body and allows it to operate optimally in both dynamic and static situations.

Body movements are executed through the contraction of muscle cells, however, as already noted, the muscular system not only moves the body but also holds and stabilizes it. A certain level of muscle tone exists at all times, and at any given moment, there will always be a few fibers in minimal action.

Anatomically, muscular functioning and design depend on the arrangement of the fibers. Muscles contain a great number of muscle fibers tied together in "bundles". Muscular activity does not activate all of these fibers: some remain "in reserve", ready for action should the muscle begin to show signs of fatigue.

Each muscle has an origin and an insertion (Fig. 2.2). In most daily functions, the origin remains fixed and the insertion is the point that moves. The main insertion of a muscle is in the bone itself, and its position is not necessarily in a straight line but on the diagonal (such as the oblique abdominal muscles), which facilitates faster action with less contraction, thus conserving energy (Baharav, 1972).

This chapter will deal with the muscular system and its posture-related functions:

- Performing movement in various parts of the body
- Maintaining joint stability
- Assisting the breathing process (mainly the diaphragm and intercostal muscles).

Muscular activity – kinesiological aspects

Because muscle action entails pulling the bones which they are attached to, the body's muscular system is arranged in a manner that wraps each joint with groups of opposing – antagonistic – muscles.

Balance between antagonistic muscle groups is absolutely essential for normal posture. Lack of balance between these muscle groups can also impair skeletal carriage and overload the lower extremity joints, the pelvis, the shoulder girdle and the spinal column (Nudelman & Reis, 1990) (Fig. 2.3).

Each movement involves a number of muscles. In each such "cooperative effort", muscular functioning can be classified as follows:

- The main muscle performing the required action (the prime mover)
- The antagonist muscle that permits the movement by relaxing
- The synergistic muscles that assist the prime move
- The "fixators" that establish a specific part of the body as a stable base from which the movement can be performed.

Muscular function also varies according to body position. Aside from creating motion, muscles can also prevent movement, therefore a distinction should be made between muscular activity in static and dynamic situations. For example, the deltoid is the main muscle responsible for (the dynamic act of) raising one's arm to the side (abduction), but the same muscle is also very important for holding that arm up (a static act) when it is already abducted (Fig. 2.4).

Thus, muscles may act in three main ways:

1. Performing a movement by means of contraction against gravity or against some other external force (concentric contraction).
2. Allowing movement by lengthening with gravity (eccentric contraction).
3. Preventing movement statically against gravity. In cases of static action, the muscle can function at a normal, shortened or extended length, depending on the nature of activity and the body position.

The role of the muscular system in maintaining posture

While the muscular system has a static function, its most basic and essential role is movement, and any static state in which the body finds itself is merely part of this basic activity. Many researchers (Kendal & McCreary, 1983; Kisner & Colby, 1985; Chukuka et al., 1986) see posture muscles as facilitating erect stature, but it should be kept in mind that under optimal physiological conditions, the maintenance of balanced standing requires very little muscular energy. Strong muscular activity indicates a postural disorder. *Note the paradox*: while posture muscles are viewed by some as enabling the body to be held static while standing, such a state actually requires very little muscular activity.

Basmajian (1978) noted this paradox and argued that only a narrow and limited definition would call normal posture that state in which the body stands straight, so that the forces acting upon it from all directions are balanced (Fig. 2.5). This definition deals only with the ability to maintain one's body in a standing position against gravity and to balance the center of gravity of each limb above the one below it. However, a broader definition must take other situations into consideration, such as sitting, lying or even walking – states that people experience in their daily activities.

In reviewing the anatomic and physiological characteristics of the body joints, this chapter will concentrate only on those aspects related directly to the posture system. Thus, it will not include all the muscles around each joint, only the main ones.

The special characteristics of each joint will be presented as follows:

- An anatomical survey of each joint's structural dictates and bones
- A survey of the main muscles affecting joint position and function
- A kinesiological survey of joint mobility for maintaining posture.

The detailed tables in this chapter (Tables 2.1–2.7) will list the names of the muscles, together with their connections to the skeletal system, in English or Latin, according to the generally accepted terminology used in the professional anatomy literature.

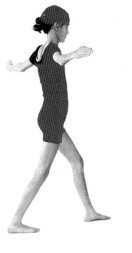

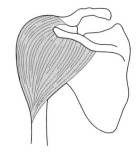

Figure 2.4 The deltoid muscle (below) and its action.

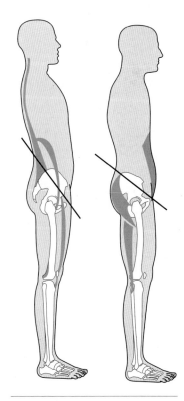

Figure 2.5 Postural muscles in a static standing position.

THE FOOT

The foot

Anatomical aspects

Because of its structure and its many connecting joints, the foot can bear the weight of the body combining optimal stability with mobility. If its structure is normal, body weight can be borne with minimum energy expenditure by the muscular system.

Because the foot also serves as a shock-absorber it must adapt itself to a variety of surfaces as it steps down in dynamic functions such as walking, running, and jumping. Even when underlying surfaces are not level (as on sand, grass, and inclines), it must adjust to conditions and provide a solid base for the structures and joints above it.

The foot bones are divided into three groups (Fig. 2.6):

1. 7 tarsals
2. 5 metatarsals
3. 14 phalanges.

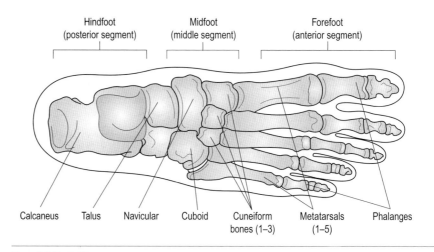

Figure 2.6 The foot bones.

Kinesiological aspects

The foot as a structure must bear a lot of weight, often much more than the weight of the body. To do this, the foot has two arches (Fig. 2.7):

- A longitudinal arch
- A transverse arch.

The normal range of these arches is of great importance for posture, as they make it possible for the foot to combine strength and stability with flexibility and springiness. Lower or higher than normal arches are disorders with potentially adverse effects on general posture (these disorders will be addressed separately in Ch. 5).

A normal foot arch depends on the anatomical position of several structures arranged along what is called the Feiss Line (Fig. 2.8) (Norkin & Levangie, 1993):

- Medial malleolus
- Navicular tuberosity
- First metatarsal head.

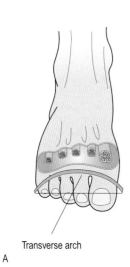

Transverse arch

A

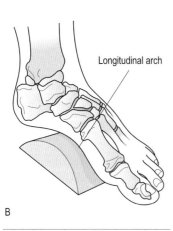

Longitudinal arch

B

Figure 2.7 Foot arches. (A) Transverse arch. (B) Longitudinal arch.

Muscles affecting the foot

Table 2.1

ORIGIN	INSERTION	ACTION	FIGURES
TIBIALIS POSTERIOR			
• Tibia: posterior lateral surface • Fibula: proximal medial surface and interosseous membrane	• Navicular tuberosity • Plantar surface of three cuneiform bones	• Plantar flexion of foot with inversion • Maintains foot arches	
FLEXOR HALLUCIS BREVIS			
• Medial cuneiform and tendon of tibialis posterior	• Through two tendons on lateral and medial side of first phalange	• Flexion of large toe • Helps to maintain foot arches	
PERONEUS LONGUS			
• Head of fibula and lateral proximal region of fibular body	• Plantar surface of 1st metatarsal and medial cuneiform	• Assists in plantar flexion with eversion • Maintains foot arches	
PERONEUS BREVIS			
• Distal lateral surface of fibula	• Base of 5th metatarsal	• Plantar flexion of foot with eversion	
PERONEUS TERTIUS			
• Distal frontal medial surface of fibula	• Dorsal side of base of 5th metatarsal	• Dorsiflexion of foot with slight eversion	

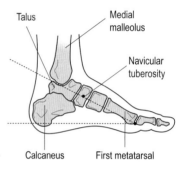

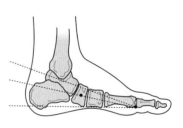

Figure 2.8 Feiss line for evaluating foot arches.

The ankle joint

Anatomical aspects

The ankle joint is formed at the meeting point of the two leg bones (tibia + fibula) with the talus (Fig. 2.9).

This joint allows dorsiflexion and plantar flexion on the sagittal plane. Normally, potential range of movement on this plane is 70°. Foot movements in the coronal/frontal plane do not occur in the ankle but rather just below it, in what is called the subtalar joint. This joint, which is formed by the talus and the calcaneus, has three articulated surfaces that permit inversion and eversion. These movements (on the frontal plane) can be performed at a range of about 60° (Kahle et al., 1986).

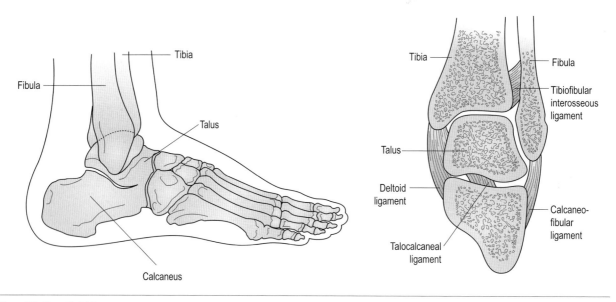

Figure 2.9 The ankle joint.

Kinesiological aspects

Albeit its relatively small dimensions, the ankle joint has an important role in posture and in transferring body weight to the foot during standing, walking, and running. Quite naturally, the ankle joint protects its stability with the assistance of leg muscle tone and a system of support ligaments arrayed in several directions.

Anatomically, the lateral malleolus is located somewhat distal and posterior to the medial malleolus. This is why the movement axis of the ankle joint is imbalanced, with a lateral tilt of about 10° (Hamilton & Luttgens, 2002).

As in all mechanisms whose parts and components are exposed to multidirectional movement, the ankle is easily injured when excessive forces are exerted on it. The joint is especially sensitive to sharp rapid changes of body movement and direction.

Muscles affecting the ankle joint

Table 2.2

ORIGIN	INSERTION	ACTION	FIGURES
GASTROCNEMIUS			
• Medial/lateral femoral condyles and knee capsule	• Through Achilles tendon to calcaneal tuberosity	• Plantar flexion of foot • Assisting in knee flexion	
SOLEUS			
• Soleal line of tibia • Medial 1/3 of tibia • Upper posterior surface of fibular head	• Calcaneal tuberosity	• Plantar flexion of foot	
PLANTARIS			
• Lateral femoral condyles • Knee capsule	• Calcaneal tuberosity	• Plantar flexion of foot • Works with soleus and gastrocnemius (triceps surae)	
TIBIALIS ANTERIOR			
• Superior lateral 2/3 of tibia	• Medial cuneiform and base of metatarsal No. 1	• Dorsiflexion of foot with slight inversion	
EXTENSOR DIGITORUM LONGUS			
• Lateral upper 1/3 of tibia • Fibular head and upper anterior surface of fibular body	• Toes 2–5	• Extension of toes 2–5 to dorsiflexion of foot	

The knee joint

Anatomical aspects

The knee is one of the most complex and vulnerable joints in the body. It is located between two long bones (the femur and tibia), and carries weight using long movement levers. This explains why such strong forces and moments are activated on it.

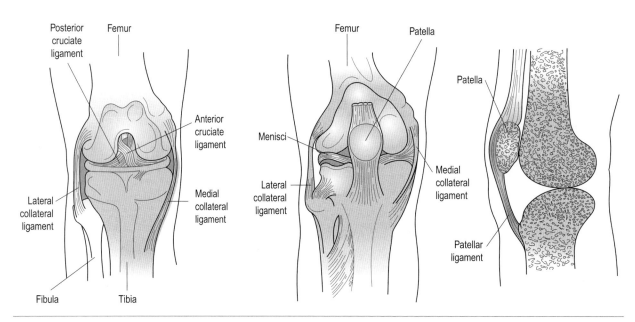

Figure 2.10 Right knee from front and side (anterior and lateral view).

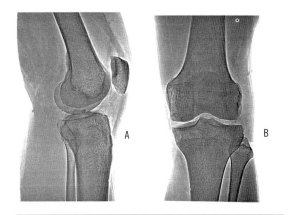

Figure 2.11 X-ray of knee joint. (A) From the side. (B) From behind.

Three joints are attached to the knee (see Fig. 2.10):

- Patella-femoral joint
- Medial tibia-femoral joint
- Lateral tibia-femoral joint

Anatomically, the flat articular surfaces of the tibia do not provide sufficient support for the thigh bone, with its semicircular (condyle) end, when direct lateral and rotational forces act on the knee. Because of this delicate and complex mechanism and despite the menisci that somewhat add to bone support, the entire joint mechanism is vulnerable (Fig. 2.11).

Muscles affecting the knee joint

Table 2.3

	ORIGIN	INSERTION	ACTION	FIGURES
QUADRICEPS FEMORIS	**RECTUS FEMORIS**			

	• The muscle has two heads:
	  a. Long head: anterior inferior iliac spine (AIIS)
	  b. Short head: supra-acetabular groove
		• Tibial tuberosity	• Knee extension
			• Long head assists in hip flexion	

	VASTUS MEDIALIS			
	• Medial lip of linea aspera	• Tibial tuberosity	• Knee extension	
	VASTUS LATERALIS			
	• Lateral surface of greater trochanter and lateral lip of linea aspera	• Tibial tuberosity	• Knee extension	
	VASTUS INTERMEDIUS			
	• Anterior surface of femur	• Tibial tuberosity	• Knee extension	
	BICEPS FEMORIS			
	• Long head: Ischial tuberosity • Short head: Inferior 1/2 of linea aspera	• Head of fibula	• Long head: Thigh extension; knee flexion and external rotation of leg • Short head: Knee flexion and external rotation of leg This is the only muscle to perform external leg rotation	

Muscles affecting the knee joint

Table 2.3

ORIGIN	INSERTION	ACTION	FIGURES
SEMITENDINOSUS			
• Ischial tuberosity	• Under medial condyle of tibia	• Thigh extension, knee flexion and internal rotation of leg	
SEMIMEMBRANOSUS			
• Ischial tuberosity	• Under medial condyle of tibia • Slightly lateral to semitendinosus tendon	• Thigh extension, knee flexion and internal rotation of leg	
SARTORIUS			
• Anterior superior iliac spine (ASIS)	• Lower medial condyle of tibia	• Thigh flexion • External thigh rotation • Knee flexion • Internal rotation of leg	
GRACILIS			
• Inferior ramus of pubis	• Medial condyle of tibia	• Thigh adduction • Assists in thigh flexion and internal rotation of leg • Helps in knee flexion	
GASTROCNEMIUS			
• Medial/lateral femoral condyles and knee capsule	• Through Achilles tendon to calcaneal tuberosity	• Plantar flexion of foot • Assisting in knee flexion	

Kinesiological aspects

The knee is one of the largest and strongest joints in the body and is involved in many regular activities of daily work and living. However, because of its structure, function, and location, the knee is highly vulnerable to injury.

The femur, the tibia and the patella are connected in a manner that permits the knee to perform flexion and extension, tibial rotation in relation to the femur and slight forward and backward sliding movements between the bones (Mitrany, 1993). The main knee movement is performed on the sagittal plane (flexion/extension), and when flexed the knee can also perform rotation (Fig. 2.12).

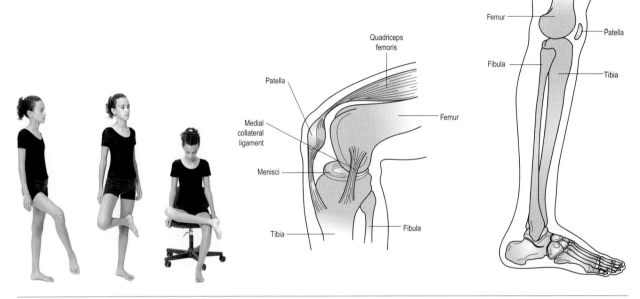

Figure 2.12 Rotation movements of the knee joint.

Functions of the patella in knee movements

The patella is a sesamoidal bone located within the tendon of the quadriceps femoris. It creates an articulated surface with the femur, which is divided into a lateral and a medial surface.

The patella helps to channel and direct the quadriceps muscle forces converging on the same point from different directions, allows concentration of forces, and assists knee extension by increasing lever arm moment (knee extension mechanism). Thus, biomechanically, the patella serves as a lever for the static and dynamic forces that develop in the knee joint (Rasch, 1989).

Kinesiologically, the patella performs movements on a number of planes, as follows:

In knee extension, the patella elevates in relation to the femoral condyles, and in knee flexion, it depresses and compresses into the femur. This sliding movement is also performed sagittally and in medial rotation. The result of these movements is that at each angle another part of the patella comes in contact with the femur (Kahle et al., 1986).

Normal functioning of the patella depends on a static and dynamic stabilization system that integrates a number of supportive ligaments and tendons. Under optimal conditions, the forces acting on the patella attain a balance (mainly on the lateral and medial sides). When this functional equilibrium is breached, the resulting malalignment of the patella position disrupts the normal movement path. The main sources of problems in this respect are usually excessive forces on the lateral side and weakness on the medial side (Kisner & Colby, 1985).

The quadriceps is the main extensor of the knee and bears the brunt of the load in many actions such as standing, walking, running, and ascending and descending steps. For knee balance to be maintained during these activities, the quadriceps must produce tremendous forces.

The knee is equipped with many ligaments that work with the muscle system to maintain joint stability during all movements, but the many synchronic movements of the various parts of the knee, together with its structural anatomical limitations, make the joint highly susceptible to injury (Mitrany, 1993). In terms of posture, a controlled and balanced movement of the femur turns the two condyles into load distributors for the joint. Correct organization of body weight and awareness of proper functioning of the knees will enable these joints to remain stable in a variety of dynamic situations. Balanced antagonistic muscle groups and normal functioning of the supportive ligaments are the main contributors to such stability (Enoka, 1994).

Measuring the Q angle of the knee joint

In addition to muscle functioning, normal position of the patella depends on anatomical structural components. One of the ways to check patellar position is by calculating the Q angle.

The Q angle is measured in relation to two lines (Fig. 2.13):

1. From the anterior superior iliac spine (ASIS) to the center of the patella and
2. From the tibial tuberosity to the center of the patella. The normative Q angle is 15°. An angle >15° increases the lateral forces working on the patella.

In order to understand the complex function of the knee, the following three axes have to be understood:

- The mechanical axis of the lower extremity
- The anatomical axes of the femur and tibia
- The movement axis.

The mechanical axis The mechanical axis of the lower extremity refers to a line that passes from the center of the head of the femur to the center of the talus. Normally, this line also passes through the center of the knee (Fig. 2.14).

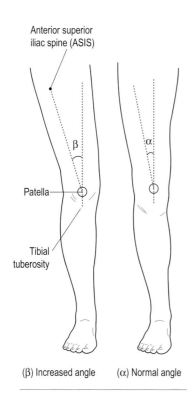

Anterior superior iliac spine (ASIS)

β

α

Patella

Tibial tuberosity

(β) Increased angle   (α) Normal angle

Figure 2.13 Measuring the Q angle.

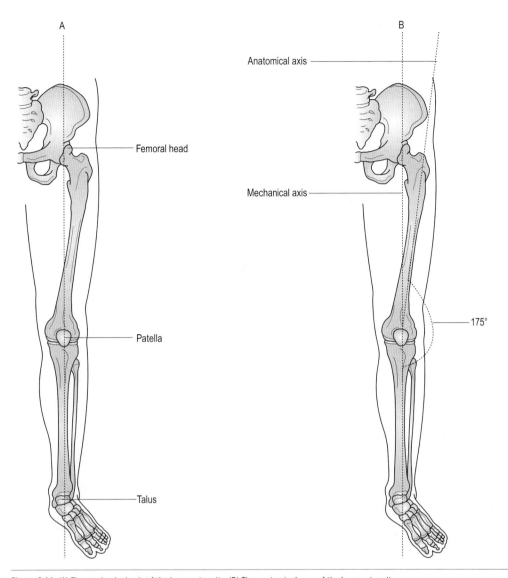

Figure 2.14 (A) The mechanical axis of the lower extremity. (B) The anatomical axes of the lower extremity.

The anatomical axis The anatomical axis refers to the line passing through the bone shaft. Usually the meeting of the anatomical axes of the femur and the tibia creates an angle (laterally) of 170–175° (the tibio-femoral angle). When this angle is <165° the result is "knock-knees" (genu valgum). When the angle is >180° the result is "bowlegs" (genu varum).

When this angle is within the normal range (Fig. 2.14B), the forces from the ground pass through the center of the knee, and loads are divided equally between the medial and lateral sides of the knee. An angle greater or lesser than the normal range exposes the knee joints to attrition and wear and tear as a result of unbalanced distributions of loads and forces acting on the joint (Steindler, 1970).

The movement axis The movement axis in knee flexion and extension traverses the femoral condyles in a straight horizontal line, changing with the range of movement along the sagittal plane.

The movement axis in rotation is a longitudinal line (through the center of the joint). When performing knee rotation in an open kinematic chain with the joint flexed at 90°, femoral-tibial joint movement is much more limited in range on the medial side than on the lateral side of the joint.

During lateral rotation, the medial plateau of the joint serves as a kind of axis for the movement. The medial tibial plateau moves very slightly forward in relation to the femoral condyle, while the lateral tibial plateau moves backwards considerably more in relation to the lateral femoral condyle (Enoka, 1994). Similarly, during medial rotation the medial part of the tibia serves as the movement axis.

Knee rotation allows a range of 70° (lateral rotation has a range of 40°, which, as noted, is somewhat more than medial rotation, the range of which can extend to 30°).

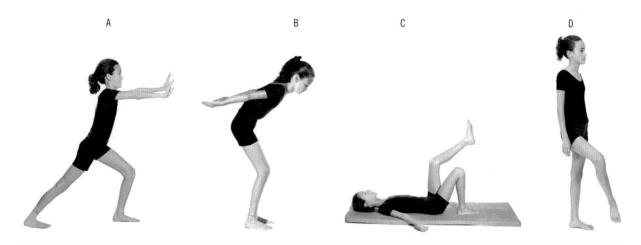

Figure 2.15 Knee movements in (A, B) a closed and (C, D) open kinematic chain.

Factors affecting range of knee movement

Knee movement in the sagittal plane (flexion and extension) is not limited mechanically by bone structure (as is the case for the elbow joint). Therefore, range of movement is determined mainly by the functioning of the joint capsule and ligaments.

As most of the muscles connected to the knee traverse two joints (the hip and knee), the range of knee movement is also dependent on hip position. Thus, for example, when the hip is in hyperextension, knee flexion will be limited by the extended state of the rectus femoris of the quadriceps, and therefore normative knee flexion ranges from 120° to 140°, depending on hip position.

In an open kinematic chain (when the leg is relaxed), the position of the hip joint will determine the range of knee movement.

In a closed kinematic chain, range of knee movement depends on the positions of both the hip and the ankle. Any functional limitation of either of these two joints (hip – ankle) will create a kinematic movement limitation of the knee as well (Hamilton & Luttgens, 2002).

Knee functioning in open kinematic chains and in closed kinematic chains

Whether a kinematic chain is open or closed affects knee movement. The lower extremities function in an open kinematic chain when the feet are off the ground. In a closed kinematic chain, the foot is in contact with the ground. The significance of the differences between open and closed kinematic chains is that in the closed chain, foot movement is limited but movement in the other joints (knee and hip) is possible.

In a closed kinematic chain, knee flexion is accompanied by hip flexion and by dorsiflexion of the ankle joint.

In an open kinematic chain, knee flexion can be performed with or without movement of the hip and ankle joints (Fig. 2.15). In Figure 2.15C, knee flexion is accompanied by hip flexion but not by ankle movement.

In open or closed kinematic chains, the functioning of the muscles acting on the knee must also be examined. For example, in knee extension in an open kinematic chain, the quadriceps is active, while in the closed kinematic chain the hamstrings and gluteus maximus also participate in straightening the knee.

THE HIP JOINT

The hip joint

Anatomical aspects

The hip joint is formed at the meeting point of the femoral head with the acetabulum in the pelvis (Fig. 2.16). In addition to the osseous structure, the joint is stabilized by a network of ligaments and a variety of muscles, which envelop it from all sides and provide a combination of power and stability with broad movement in all planes.

Muscles affecting the hip joint

Table 2.4

	ORIGIN	INSERTION	ACTION	FIGURES
ILIOPSOAS — **PSOAS MAJOR**	• Sides of the lumbar vertebrae and side of T12	• Lesser trochanter	• Thigh flexion with some external rotation • Increasing lumbar lordosis	
ILIACUS	• Superior 2/3 of anterior surface in iliac fossa	• Lesser trochanter of femur	• Thigh flexion • Anterior pelvic tilt and increasing lumbar lordosis	
GLUTEUS MAXIMUS	• Iliac crest • Posterior superior iliac spine (PSIS) • Sacrum	• Gluteal tuberosity	• Thigh extension and external rotation • Posterior pelvic tilt • As the connection point of the muscle is spread over a large area, the muscle can also help in both thigh abduction and adduction (depending on which fibers contract)	
GLUTEUS MEDIUS	• Gluteal surface of ilium (between the posterior and anterior gluteal line on the ilium bone)	• Greater trochanter	• Anterior fibers: Internal rotation and thigh flexion • Posterior fibers: External rotation and thigh extension • General contraction of the muscle creates thigh abduction • Standing on one leg prevents prolapse of the pelvis on the side of the supporting leg (Trendelenburg syndrome)	

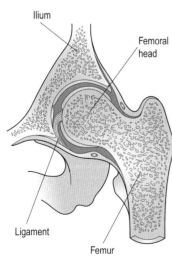

Ilium

Femoral head

Ligament

Femur

Figure 2.16 The hip joint.

Muscles affecting the hip joint

Table 2.4

ORIGIN	INSERTION	ACTION	FIGURES
PIRIFORMIS			
• Anterior surface of sacrum between the 1st and 4th foramen • Greater sciatic notch	• Anteromedial aspect of the tip of the greater trochanter	• External rotation of thigh • Assists in thigh abduction	
OBTURATOR INTERNUS			
• Inner surface of the pubis around the obturator foramen • Ischium	• Anteromedial aspect of the greater trochanter	• External rotation of thigh	
OBTURATOR EXTERNUS			
• External surface of the obturator foramen and the obturator membrane • Ramus of ischium	• Medial aspect of greater trochanter of femur	• External rotation of thigh	
GEMELLUS SUPERIOR			
• Ischial spine	• Medial aspect of greater trochanter	• External rotation of thigh	
GEMELLUS INFERIOR			
• Ischial tuberosity	• Medial aspect of greater trochanter	• External rotation of thigh	

*Most of the muscles whose origin is in the pelvic region connect to the femur.

Other muscles working on the hip joint will be detailed later in this chapter (Table 2.5, Muscles affecting the pelvis).

Muscles affecting the hip joint

Table 2.4

ORIGIN	INSERTION	ACTION	FIGURES
PECTINEUS			
• Pubic tubercle	• Pectineal line behind lesser trochanter of femur	• Thigh flexion • Thigh adduction • Internal rotation of thigh	
ADDUCTOR BREVIS			
• Inferior ramus of pubis	• Superior 1/3 of linea aspera	• Thigh adduction • External rotation of thigh • Assists in thigh flexion	
ADDUCTOR LONGUS			
• Superior ramus of pubis	• Middle 1/3 of the medial lip of linea aspera	• Thigh adduction • Assists in thigh flexion • External rotation of thigh	
ADDUCTOR MAGNUS			
• Anterior surface of the inferior ramus of the pubis • Inferior ramus of ischium and ischial tuberosity	• Muscle fibers are divided in two: Horizontal (anterior) fibers: Along linea aspera Vertical (posterior) fibers: Adductor tubercle slightly above medial epicondyle	• Thigh adduction • Horizontal fibers (connected to linea aspera) create external rotation • Vertical fibers create medial rotation (from a state of lateral rotation when lower extremity is flexed) • Vertical fibers also create thigh extension	
ADDUCTOR MINIMUS			
• Inferior ramus of pubis	• Linea aspera	• Thigh adduction • External thigh rotation	

Kinesiological aspects

The hip joint allows movement on all three planes:

- Flexion–extension on the sagittal plane
- Abduction–adduction on the frontal/coronal plane
- External rotation–internal rotation on the horizontal plane
- Circumduction on all planes.

Normative movement ranges for the hip joint vary according to joint position of the neighboring knee and pelvis, and muscle length. Normative ranges in a standing anatomical position are as follows (Norkin & Levangie, 1993):

- Flexion (when the knee is flexed): 110°
- Extension: 30°
- Abduction: 50°
- Adduction: 30°
- Lateral rotation: 60°
- Medial rotation: 40°.

The normative range for lateral hip rotation is 60°, which is more than the 40° attained in medial rotation (in a sitting position when the joint is flexed, hip rotation is somewhat greater because the joint capsule and ligaments are freer).

Functional balance between the antagonistic muscle groups acting on the hip joint is a precondition for normal position of the lower extremities (below) and the pelvis (above).

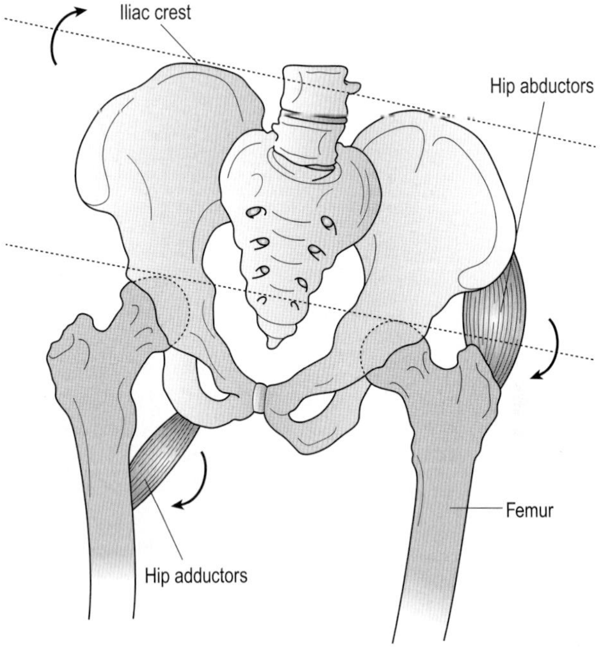

Figure 2.17 Deviation of the pelvic position due to lack of balance in antagonistic muscle groups (shortening of the adductors).

On the frontal plane, the hip adductors on one side act as synergists with the abductors on the other side. Normally, the adductors and abductors apply equal forces from both sides, but lack of balance in these forces will cause a deviation in the hip position (Nordin & Frankel, 1989).

A shortening of the hip adductors or abductors is one cause of hip imbalance. A shortening of the adductors will elevate the hip on that side, which may give the appearance of unequal leg length (Fig. 2.17).

Horizontal plane balance depends on a functional balance between the muscle groups surrounding the hip inside and out. As most of the muscles connecting the hip to the femur facilitate external rotation, the force of the muscles rotating internally is smaller than that of external rotation. A greater than normal differential in this force ratio is reflected in excessive force in external hip rotation, which is one of the causes of toe-out position (other causes will be discussed in Ch. 5).

THE PELVIS

The pelvis
Anatomical aspects

The position of the pelvis in the center of the body creates a functional chain effect on both the lower extremities and on the position of the spinal column. The normal functioning of the pelvis is made possible by maintenance of a functional balance between movement ability and stability, which is provided by muscular action. The connection of the spinal column to the pelvis creates the "pelvic angle" (Fig. 2.19).

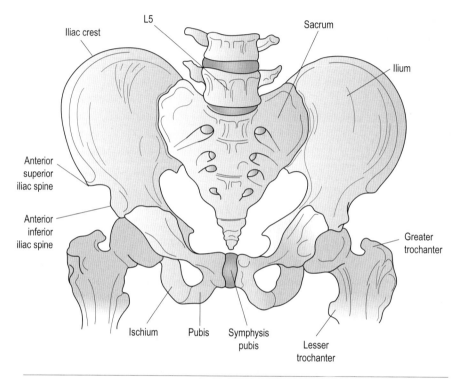

Figure 2.18 The pelvis.

This natural angle of the pelvis is usually 55° among men and 60° among women. Increasing the pelvic angle beyond the norm is one of the characteristics of increased lordosis, and lessening the incline angle reduces lumbar lordosis (Kendal & McCreary, 1983).

Pelvic balance at the optimal angle depends mainly on the normal functioning of the various muscles. The lower part of the back erectors, together with the rectus femoris of the thigh and with the iliopsoas muscles, turn the pelvis forward, that is, they increase the incline angle and the lumbar lordosis in the spinal column. In the opposite direction the three hamstrings together with the abdominal muscles and the gluteus maximus perform posterior pelvic tilt, that is, they decrease the incline angle and thus lessen lordosis in the lumbar vertebrae (Fig. 2.20).

Normal posture on the lumbar sagittal plane depends, in part, on coordination among all of these muscles. The aim of remedial exercise is to train individuals to "feel" the right relationship in the activity of these muscles, and where necessary to improve the balance in their functioning.

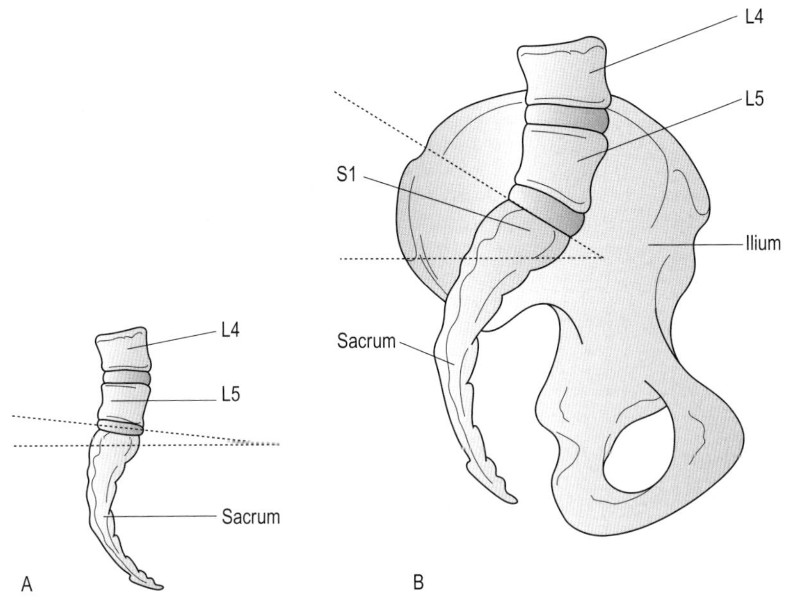

Figure 2.19 Meeting point of the sacrum and the spinal column (L5–S1). (A) A decreased angle. (B) A normal angle.

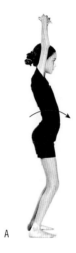

The sacrum

The connection point of the lumbar spinal column to the sacrum is a sensitive focus for the creation of loads in daily functioning. These pressures are reflected in the high frequency of injuries to the intervertebral discs at the meeting point L5–S1 (Fig. 2.19) (Cyriax, 1979; Kisner & Colby, 1985; Kahle et al., 1986).

The connection of the sacrum to the pelvis creates another important joint – the sacroiliac joint – which facilitates a minor sliding movement in a number of planes (Fig. 2.21). The movements of the sacrum in relation to the ilium depend on the mobility of the spinal column in the way in which in positions of flexion the sacrum moves posteriorly and in torso extension (backwards), the sacrum moves forward.

Kinesiologically, the sacrum is affected mainly by the movements created in the torso, and it responds accordingly (bending the torso forward creates sacrum movement to the rear and vice versa).

On the other hand, the iliac bones in the pelvis are affected mainly by hip movement; therefore, it can be said that the position of the sacrum depends on the forces acting on it from above, while the position of the iliac bones depends mainly on the forces acting on them from below.

In movements performed in a closed kinematic chain, sacrum position is affected by forces acting on it from below as well (Rasch, 1989).

Ilium movement in relation to the sacrum is essential for balance in the static and dynamic position of the spinal column and of the lower extremities. Functional disorders in the sacroiliac joint can cause movement fixation, and in time they can also cause postural disorders.

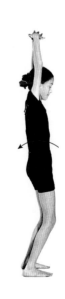

Figure 2.20 Pelvic mobility in (A) anterior and (B) posterior tilt.

THE PELVIS

Muscles affecting the pelvis

Table 2.5

	ORIGIN	INSERTION	ACTION	FIGURES
PSOAS MAJOR				
ILIOPSOAS	• Sides of the lumbar vertebrae and side of T12	• Lesser trochanter	• Thigh flexion with some external rotation • Increasing lumbar lordosis	
ILIACUS				
	• Superior 2/3 of anterior surface in iliac fossa	• Lesser trochanter of femur	• Thigh flexion • Anterior pelvic tilt and increasing lumbar lordosis	
PSOAS MINOR				
	• Sides of vertebrae T12–L1	• The point of connection between the iliacus and upper ramus of pubis	• Flexion of torso to pelvis	
GLUTEUS MAXIMUS				
	• Iliac crest • Posterior superior iliac spine (PSIS) • Sacrum	• Gluteal tuberosity	• Thigh extension and external rotation • Posterior pelvic tilt • As the connection point of the muscle is spread over a large area, the muscle can also help in both thigh abduction and adduction (depending on which fibers contract)	
GLUTEUS MEDIUS				
	• Gluteal surface of ilium (between the posterior and anterior gluteal line on the ilium bone)	• Greater trochanter	• Anterior fibers: Internal rotation and thigh flexion • Posterior fibers: External rotation and thigh extension • General contraction of the muscle creates thigh abduction • Standing on one leg prevents prolapse of the pelvis on the side of the supporting leg (Trendelenburg syndrome)	

Muscles affecting the pelvis

Table 2.5

ORIGIN	INSERTION	ACTION	FIGURES
GLUTEUS MINIMUS			
• Surface between anterior and inferior gluteal lines on the ilium	• Greater trochanter	• Abduction and internal rotation of thigh	
TENSOR FASCIA LATA			
• Anterior superior iliac spine (ASIS) and continues above greater trochanter along the iliotibial tract	• Lateral tibial condyle	• Stabilizes femur head in the acetabulum • Assists anterior fibers of gluteus minimus and medius in thigh flexion, internal rotation and abduction	
SARTORIUS			
• Anterior superior iliac spine (ASIS)	• Lower medial condyle of tibia	• Thigh flexion • External thigh rotation • Knee flexion • Internal rotation of leg	
SEMITENDINOSUS			
• Ischial tuberosity	• Under medial condyle of tibia	• Thigh extension, knee flexion and internal rotation of leg	
SEMIMEMBRANOSUS			
• Ischial tuberosity	• Under medial condyle of tibia • Slightly lateral to semitendinosus tendon	• Thigh extension, knee flexion and internal rotation of leg	

THE PELVIS

Muscles affecting the pelvis

Table 2.5

ORIGIN	INSERTION	ACTION	FIGURES
BICEPS FEMORIS			
• Long head: Ischial tuberosity • Short head: Inferior 1/2 of linea aspera	• Head of fibula	• Long head: Thigh extension; Knee flexion and external rotation of leg • Short head: Knee flexion and external rotation of leg This is the only muscle to perform external leg rotation	
GRACILIS			
• Inferior ramus of pubis	• Medial condyle of tibia	• Thigh adduction • Assists in thigh flexion and internal rotation of leg • Helps in knee flexion	
QUADRATUS LUMBORUM			
• Rib No. 12 • Transverse processes of lumbar vertebra L1–4	• Iliac crest	• Helps in anterior pelvic tilt and increasing lumbar lordosis • When the pelvis is fixed, it helps in raising the torso to erect from a state of forward flexion • Helps in side flexion	
RECTUS ABDOMINIS			
• Two sides of sternum and cartilage of ribs 5–7	• Superior ramus of pubis	• Flexion of thoracic cage and pelvis towards each other, and thus straightening of lumbar lordosis in posterior pelvic tilt • In unilateral action on one side, helps with side flexion of torso	
EXTERNAL ABDOMINAL OBLIQUE			
• Ribs 5–12	• The fibers beginning at the lower ribs connect to the iliac crest • Rest of muscle fibers connect to aponeurosis	• Helps in side flexion of torso	

Kinesiological aspects

In daily functioning, pelvic mobility occurs in a few movement planes, depending on which joints are involved (Figs 2.21, 2.22). Functionally, movements in the pelvis are possible in three planes:

1. The sagittal plane – anterior/posterior pelvic tilt (APT/PPT)
2. The frontal plane – elevation and depression of iliac crest
3. The horizontal plane – leading one side forward and backward.

Because of the chain principle and the complex functional structure of the spinal column, movement of the pelvis usually affects a few vertebrae in the lumbar region, and is not focused only on the point of connection, L5-S1.

The structure of the pelvis allows us to bear weight, but kinesiologically, as in the shoulder girdle, the pelvis also facilitates an increase in the range of hip joint movement. Rotation in the pelvis makes stepping forward possible in walking, and side flexion of the pelvis permits the lower extremity to be elevated laterally in abduction. Since pelvic position affects the organization of posture, it is important to examine whether it is fully balanced in terms of placement in all three planes. Two main factors are involved:

1. Functional balance of the length and strength ratios between the antagonistic muscles that are connected to it and affect its stabilization. This balance is especially important in the ratio between the abdominal muscles, the gluteals, and the hamstrings, which tilt the pelvis posteriorly, and on the other side, the lower erector spinae, the iliopsoas, the quadriceps (rectus femoris), and the sartorius, which tilt the pelvis anteriorly (Fig. 2.22). Shortening or weakening of the soft tissues that connect to the pelvis may upset this balance (Kendal & MacCreary, 1983; Kisner & Colby, 1985).

2. Individuals' awareness of the proper location of the pelvis and the kinesthetic ability to maintain this balance in daily activities (this aspect will be dealt with in greater detail in Ch. 9).

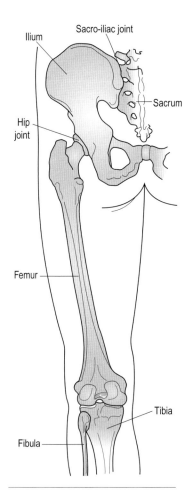

Figure 2.21 Connection of pelvis at the hip joint.

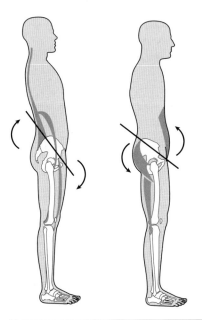

Figure 2.22 Muscles affecting pelvic position.

The spinal column

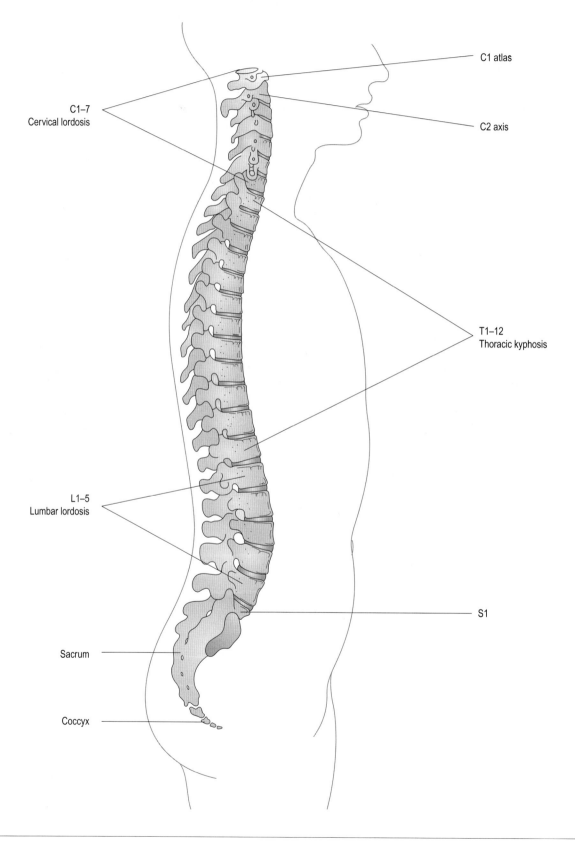

C1 atlas

C1–7
Cervical lordosis

C2 axis

T1–12
Thoracic kyphosis

L1–5
Lumbar lordosis

S1

Sacrum

Coccyx

Figure 2.23 Spinal column: views from the side, front, and back.

THE SPINAL COLUMN

Anatomical aspects

The functional relationships among the articulated surfaces in the vertebrae, the intervertebral discs, the muscles, the ligaments, and the nervous system create a complex system. This complexity constitutes a challenge to therapists both in diagnosis and in developing an adapted exercise program.

Correct diagnosis and adapted movement treatment entail an understanding of characteristic anatomical and kinesiological aspects of the spinal column. Understanding the structural dictates that affect potential movements of the various areas of the spinal column is a precondition for the proper planning of exercises and for avoiding injury.

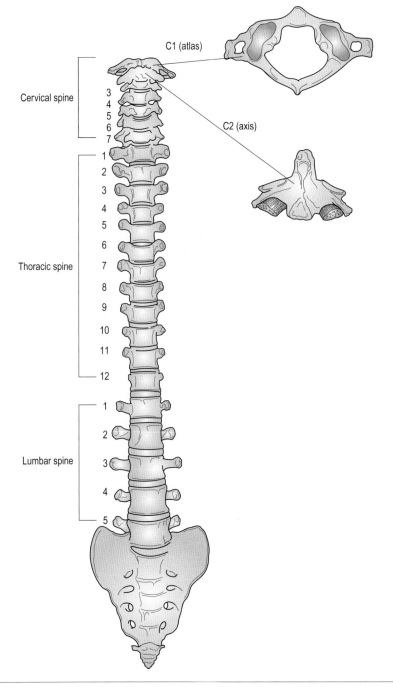
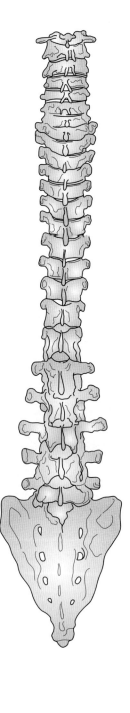

Figure 2.23 (*continued*).

The general structure of a typical vertebra in the spinal column (Fig. 2.24): The vertebra has two main parts:

- The vertebral body
- The neural arch.

Between the vertebral body and neural arch is the vertebral foramen. The neural arch has several important structures:

- The spinous process
- The transverse process
- The articular process.

Cervical verterbrae

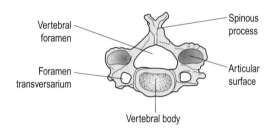

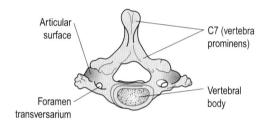

Lateral view

Superior view

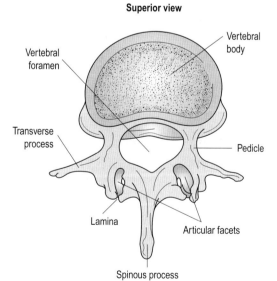

Figure 2.24 General structure of the vertebra.

Special anatomical characteristics of different areas of the spinal column

When looking at the entire skeleton, spinal curves are easily visible (Fig. 2.23):

- Cervical lordosis (C1–C7)
- Thoracic kyphosis (T1–12)
- Lumbar lordosis (L1–5).

The vertebrae in each of the spinal areas have unique characteristic traits that dictate their movement options. These traits gradually blur at the meeting point of two areas.

Main movement planes of the spinal column

C1–7 Cervical area (Fig. 2.25)

- Movement on the horizontal plane (turning head from side to side between vertebrae C1-2)
- Movement on the frontal plane (side flexing of the cervical vertebrae; lowering ear to shoulder)
- Movement on the sagittal plane (flexion and extension).

T1–12 Thoracic area (Fig. 2.26)

- Movement on the frontal plane (side flexion of the torso)
- Movement on the horizontal plane (spinal rotation).

Because of the osseous structure of these vertebrae and their connection to the rib cage of the chest, ranges of motion in this area are limited and most of the movements described involve other joints in the lumbar and cervical areas.

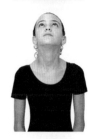
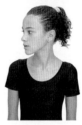
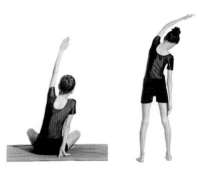

Figure 2.25 Possible movements of the cervical vertebrae.

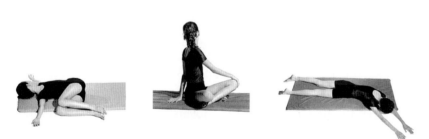
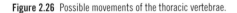

Figure 2.26 Possible movements of the thoracic vertebrae.

L1–5 Lumbar area (Fig. 2.27)

- In these vertebrae, the main movement is possible in the sagittal plane (flexion and extension of the lower back).

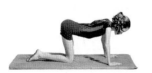
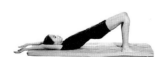
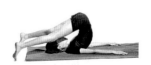

Figure 2.27 Possible movements of the lumbar vertebrae.

THE SPINAL COLUMN

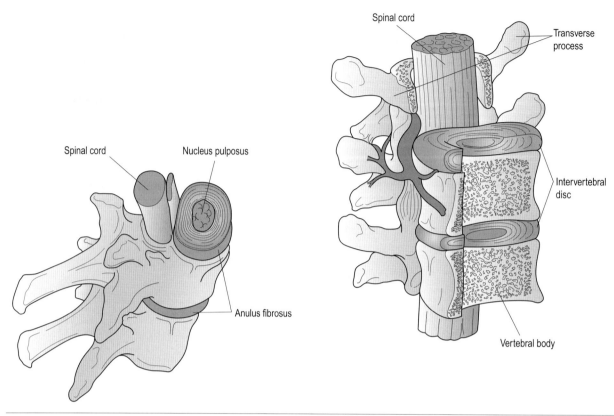

Figure 2.28 The intervertebral disc.

The intervertebral disc

The intervertebral disc serves as a point for support and for transferring loads between the vertebrae. It allows movement between the vertebrae and helps to absorb shocks along the entire spinal column. Intervertebral discs have two main structures (Fig. 2.28):

- Nucleus pulposus – a gel-like substance composed mainly of protein material and water
- Anulus fibrosus – the external part of the disc, composed of rigid connective tissue containing collagen.

Structural or functional disorders in the spinal column expose the intervertebral discs to degenerative changes. These processes, the result of attrition over the years, reduce the discs' capacity to bear mechanical loads and cause injuries such as slipped or protruding discs (see Ch. 3).

Spinal column ligaments

The function of the ligaments is to stabilize the spinal column and limit its movement on the various planes. The main ligaments along the length of the spinal column are: (see Figs 2.29, 2.30, 2.31)

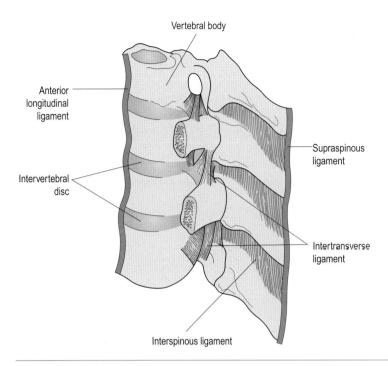

Figure 2.29 Spinal ligaments – from the side.

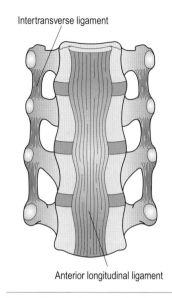

Figure 2.30 Spinal ligaments – from the front.

- Anterior longitudinal ligament – which traverses the length of the vertebrae on their anterior side. This ligament limits body movement to the rear
- Posterior longitudinal ligament – which traverses posterior to the vertebral bodies in the vertebral foramen. This ligament passes and touches each vertebra and constitutes the anterior wall of the spinal column canal
- Ligamenta flava serves as the posterior wall of the spinal column canal
- Interspinous ligament passes between one spinous process to the next and limits posterior spinal extension and anterior torso flexion
- Supraspinous ligament passes through the posterior spinous processes and limits anterior flexion of the body
- Intertransversarii ligament passes between the transverse processes in the spinal vertebrae and limits torso movement in side flexion in the frontal plane.

The deep back muscles that stabilize the spinal column (erector spinae)

The muscles in the deep erector spinae group are required to work constantly against the force of gravity, and they facilitate spinal movement and stability.

Anatomically, the erector spinae are arranged on both sides of the spinal column, from the center out. These muscles can be classified into two groups:

- The lateral-superficial group (which traverses the back from the pelvis to the skull)
- The medial-deep group (in which some of the muscles are arranged longitudinally-straight, and some obliquely).

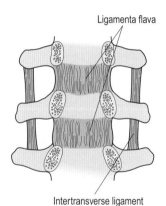

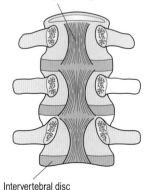

Figure 2.31 Longitudinal cross-section of the spinal column.

Muscles affecting the spinal column

The lateral (superficial) group are divided into three groups

Table 2.6a

ILIOCOSTALIS		
ILIOCOSTALIS LUMBORUM (LUMBAR REGION) • Origin in sacrum and iliac crest; insertion in the lumbar vertebrae and ribs 6–9	• The general function of all the muscles in this (lateral) group focuses mainly on body erectness and on maintaining erect posture	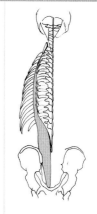
ILIOCOSTALIS THORACIS (THORACIC REGION) • Origin in bottom six ribs, insertion in the six top ribs		
ILIOCOSTALIS CERVICIS (CERVICAL REGION) • Origin in ribs 3–6 and insertion in the transverse processes of cervical vertebrae C4–6		
LONGISSIMUS		
LONGISSIMUS THORACIS (THORACIC REGION) • Origin in the sacrum, the posterior spinous processes of the lumbar vertebrae and the transverse processes of the lower thoracic vertebrae; insertion along the chest rib cage up to ribs 1–2	• Like the iliocostalis group, the function of the muscles in this group also focuses on body erectness	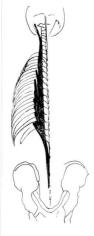
LONGISSIMUS CERVICIS (CERVICAL REGION) • Origin in the transverse processes of thoracic vertebrae T1–6 and insertion in cervical vertebrae C2–5		
LONGISSIMUS CAPITIS (HEAD REGION) • Origin in transverse processes of the thoracic vertebrae T1–5 and cervical vertebrae C4–7; insertion in the mastoid process of the skull		
SPLENIUS (INTERNAL MUSCLES)		
SPLENIUS CERVICIS (CERVICAL REGION) • Origin at the spinous processes of the thoracic vertebrae T3–6 and insertion in the transverse processes of cervical vertebrae C1–2	• The muscles in this group also function mainly in maintaining erect posture • The splenius muscles also create rotation (turning the head) when they work on one side (unilateral contraction)	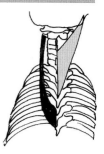
SPLENIUS CAPITIS (HEAD REGION) • Origin at the posterior spinous processes of the thoracic vertebrae T1–3 and the cervical vertebrae C4–7 and insertion at the skull in the mastoid process		

Muscles affecting the spinal column

Medial (deep) group are divided into two groups

Table 2.6b

INTERSPINALES (BETWEEN THE SPINAL PROCESSES)		
INTERSPINALES CERVICIS (CERVICAL REGION) • Six on each side **INTERSPINALES THORACIS** (THORACIC REGION) • Four on each side **INTERSPINALES LUMBORUM** (LUMBAR REGION) • Five on each side	• This group connects the vertebrae themselves, between one spinous process and the next directly (according to their location in three areas detailed)	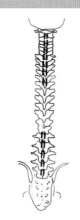
INTERTRANSVERSARII (BETWEEN THE TRANSVERSE SPINAL PROCESSES)		
INTERTRANSVERSARII CERVICIS (CERVICAL) • Six on each side **INTERTRANSVERSARII LUMBORUM** (LUMBAR) • Four on each side	• This group passes laterally to the interspinales muscles and connects in a straight line transverse process to transverse process in the spinal columm (according to their location in the two areas detailed)	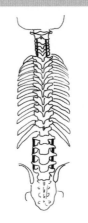
SPINALIS		
SPINALIS THORACIS (THORACIC REGION) • Origin in the spinous processes of L3 to T10 and insertion in the spinous processes of vertebrae T2–8 • The fibers are shortest between vertebrae T8–10 **SPINALIS CERVICIS** (CERVICAL REGION) Origin in the spinous processes of T2 to C6; insertion in the spinous processes of vertebrae C2–4	• These muscles pass in the thoracic and cervical areas and connect spinous process to spinous process (as they skip a few vertebrae, and not directly from one vertebra to the next)	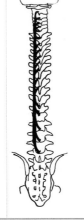

MUSCLES THAT ARE ARRANGED LONGITUDINALLY – STRAIGHT

THE SPINAL COLUMN

Muscles affecting the spinal column

Medial–deep group

Table 2.6c

ROTATORES (CREATE ROTATION)

- The muscles in this group pass along the spinal column and connect the transverse process of a given vertebra to the spinous process of the vertebra above it

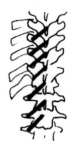

MULTIFIDUS

- This muscle is composed of many small muscles that begin in the sacral area and continue up to the neck vertebrae
- In most cases, each small muscle begins in the area of the *transverse process* of a given vertebra, skips 2–4 vertebrae and then connects to the *spinous process* of one of the vertebrae above

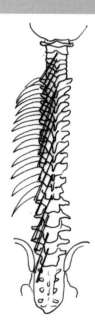

SEMISPINALIS

- These muscles pass above the multifidus on the lateral side of the thoracic, cervical and head areas:

  - Semispinalis thoracis
  - Semispinalis cervicis
  - Semispinalis capitis

- Each muscle in this group skips five vertebrae and more as it connects *transverse process* to *spinous process* in one of the vertebrae above it

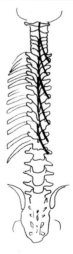

MUSCLES THAT ARE ARRANGED OBLIQUELY

*Muscle action at the deep level:

- The muscles in the group that crosses in a straight line work mainly in straightening the back and in posterior extension of the back (when two sides work together). In unilateral contraction (one side), they create sideways flexion of the torso.
- The oblique muscles work as rotators (when one side contracts they turn the torso on the horizontal plane). When both sides contract (bilateral contraction) they create posterior extension of the back.

Kinesiological aspects

The complex structure of the spinal column affords broad movement in the various planes. This movement is the sum of the small partial movements occurring between the vertebrae in keeping with the chain principle. For this reason, general mobility of the spinal column is dependent on the normal mobile functioning of the dozens of small joints between the vertebrae themselves. A local limitation directly affects range of movement in that area, and indirectly affects other areas above and below it (Steindler, 1970; Kahle et al., 1986).

As a result of chain reactions, the spinal column is also affected by the movement functioning of other structures connected to it:

- The pelvis, which attaches to the lower end of the spinal column
- The thorax, which attaches to the vertebrae in the thoracic area. It has movement potential, mainly between the ribs and the vertebrae (the costovertebral joints) and between the ribs themselves (movement seen in respiratory processes) (Kahle et al., 1986).

An understanding of these structures sharpens awareness of the complex functional ties of the skeletal system in kinesiological terms, as mobility in each joint exerts indirect mobility effects on various areas of the body, including the spinal column. These interrelationships hint at the potential for releasing and relieving many back problems through movements of the hip, pelvis or thoracic joints (discussion of this therapeutic principle appears in greater detail in Ch. 9).

Head and neck alignment

A balanced position of the head and neck is an important factor course for the organization of posture. Extended periods of incorrect positioning of the cervical vertebrae create high muscle tone in the neck extensors, which in time might also have an adverse effect on nervous structures traversing the area. Problems of this type are usually characterized by headaches, disruption of normal neural flow towards the hands, and sometimes even disruptions of normal blood flow. These disorders usually cause feelings of unease, tension, fatigue and frequent pains in the neck area (Steindler, 1970; Rasch, 1989).

Kinesiologically, there is an interrelationship between the alignment of the head and neck vertebrae and the body joints below, such as the lower extremities, the pelvis and the spinal column (Fig. 2.32). Movement therapy processes addressing head and neck tilt may create situations in which treatment for improving head tilt indirectly helps to improve lower areas as well (the shoulder girdle, the chest cage, the lower back), or conversely, treatment focusing on lower body joints may have a positive effect on head tilt. Choosing the aspects to emphasize in movement therapy depends on each patient's unique kinesiological posture characteristics, which vary from person to person.

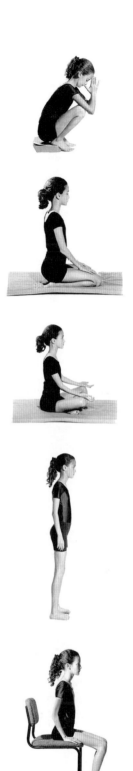

Figure 2.32 Neck position in different starting positions.

The rib cage

Anatomical aspects

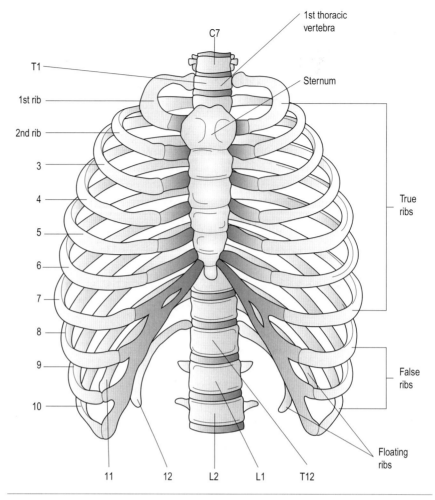

Figure 2.33 The thoracic cage.

Anatomically, the osseous thoracic or chest cage is a frame containing the 12 thoracic vertebrae of the spinal column, T1–12, 12 pairs of ribs and the sternum (Fig. 2.33). The main functions of the rib cage are:

- To protect the internal systems (heart and lungs, large blood vessels and nerves)
- To provide an anchor point for many muscles
- To actively help in the breathing process.

The first seven ribs are connected directly to the sternum by means of cartilage and are called "true ribs".

Ribs 8, 9 and 10 are connected by means of cartilage to rib 7 and are called "false ribs".

Ribs 11–12, which are called "floating ribs", are not connected to the sternum.

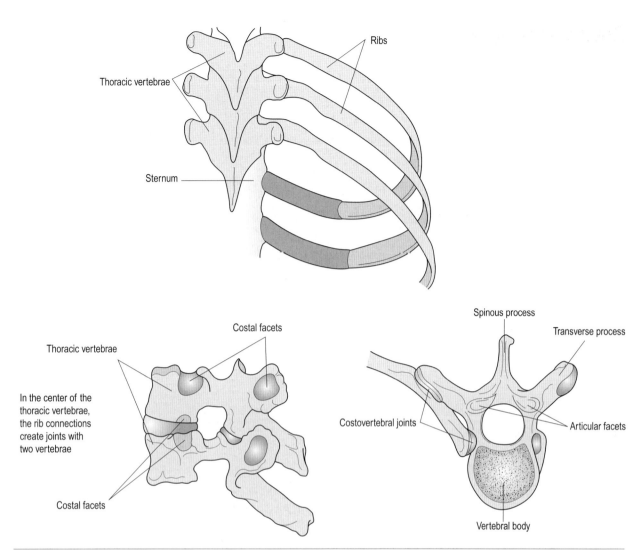

Figure 2.34 Rib cage and thoracic vertebrae.

Kinesiological aspects

The ribs create a number of joints as they connect to the sternum and to the vertebrae. Two of these joints are especially important functionally:

- The costovertebral joint (Fig. 2.34)
- The sternocostal joint.

As far as the functioning of the internal body systems is concerned, optimal thoracic cage structure and movement have a direct effect on the respiratory process. Thus, breathing is functionally related to the many joints connected to the thoracic cage area. Among them are joints connecting to the back vertebrae, joints between the ribs and vertebrae T1–12, and joints bonding ribs and sternum. The normal movement and functioning of these joints are important for maintaining optimal respiratory ranges, and movement limitations on them of any kind (such as in cases of kyphosis – see Ch. 3) will adversely affect breathing function, again indicating the connection between posture traits and functioning of the internal systems.

THE SHOULDER GIRDLE

The shoulder girdle

Anatomical aspects

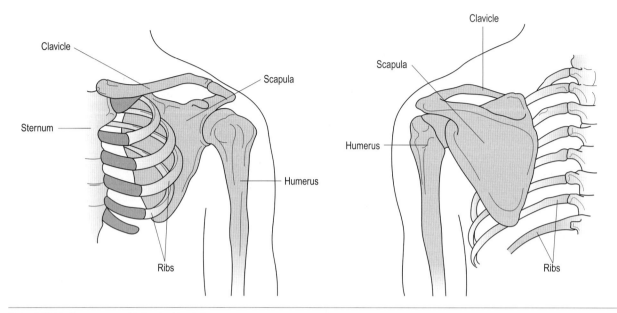

Figure 2.35 The bones connected to the shoulder girdle.

The bones connected to the shoulder girdle include the scapula, the clavicle, the rib cage, and the humerus (Fig. 2.35).

The shoulder girdle is composed of four joints that work harmoniously and synchronically, contributing to a broad range of movement in three movement planes (White & Carmeli, 1999):

- Glenohumeral joint, situated at the connection between the humerus head and the scapula. This ball and socket joint allows movement in three planes. It is enwrapped in a cartilaginous ring, reinforced by means of many ligaments and stabilized with the assistance of the rotator cuff group, and the long head of the biceps brachii (Kendall & McCreary, 1983)
- Acromioclavicular joint, situated at the connection between the apex of the scapula and the lateral end of the clavicle. This synovial joint allows circumduction in a number of planes
- Sternoclavicular joint, situated at the connecting point of the sternum and the medial end of the clavicle. This joint serves as the sole connecting point between the upper extremity and the torso
- Scapulothoracic articulation, situated at the meeting point of the scapula and the thoracic cage. Many muscles whose insertions are in the scapula, the spinal column and the arm work on this area.

Muscles affecting the shoulder girdle

Table 2.7

ORIGIN	INSERTION	ACTION	FIGURES
TRAPEZIUS			
• Superior head: Nuchal ligament and external occipital protuberance • Middle head: Spinous processes of vertebrae C7–T4 • Inferior head: Spinous processes of vertebrae T5–12	• Superior head: Lateral 1/3 of clavicle • Middle head: Spine of scapula and acromion • Inferior head: Spine of scapula	• Whole-muscle action: creates scapular adduction • Upper fibers: Scapular rotation, scapular elevation, and head extension posteriorly • Lower fibers: Scapular rotation and scapular depression In its static function the muscle stabilizes the scapula in the shoulder girdle	
LEVATOR SCAPULAE			
• Dorsal tubercles of transverse processes of vertebrae C1–4	• Superior angle of scapula and adjacent part of the medial margin	• Elevation and medial rotation of scapula • In opposite action: flexes the neck laterally and turns it to same side	
RHOMBOIDEUS MINOR			
• Spinous processes of vertebrae C6–7	• Medial margin of scapula	• Scapular adduction with some elevation • Affixing scapulae to thoracic cage	
RHOMBOIDEUS MAJOR			
• Spinous processes of vertebrae T1–4	• Along medial (vertebral) border of scapula (under rhomboideus minor)	• Scapular adduction • Affixing scapulae to thoracic cage	

The scapula is the attachment point for many muscles, and it facilitates optimal free functioning for movements of the upper extremity.

Unlike the stable structure of the hip joint, the anatomical structure of the shoulder joint is more vulnerable. The rotator cuff muscles have the important function of maintaining joint stability and compressing the humerus head into the scapular hollow (Hoppenfeld, 1976).

The rotator cuff contains the following muscles: supraspinatus, infraspinatus, subscapularis, teres minor.
*Details of the specific actions of each muscle in this group are described below.

THE SHOULDER GIRDLE

Muscles affecting the shoulder girdle

Table 2.7

ORIGIN	INSERTION	ACTION	FIGURES
DELTOIDEUS			
• Anterior clavicular head: Lateral third of clavicle • Medial-scapular head: Acromion • Posterior-scapular head: Lower border of scapular spine	• Deltoid tuberosity on lateral superior 1/3 of humerus	• Arm abduction beyond 30° (clavicular head and posterior scapular head help in arm adduction) • Anterior muscle fibers also perform internal rotation from a position in which the arm is rotated externally • Posterior muscle fibers also perform external rotation from a position in which the arm is rotated internally	
SUPRASPINATUS			
• Medial 2/3 of supraspinous fossa	• Superior surface of greater tubercle of humerus	• Arm abduction 0–30° with slight lateral rotation • Stabilizes humerus head in shoulder joint	
INFRASPINATUS			
• Medial 2/3 of infraspinous fossa	• Greater tubercle of humerus	• External rotation of humerus and arm extension • Stabilizes humerus head in shoulder joint	
SERRATUS ANTERIOR			
• Ribs 1–9 near connecting point of osseous part to cartilage	• Along vertebral (medial) margin of scapula	• Holds the vertebral ridge of the scapula to thoracic cage (together with rhomboid muscles) • In opposite action (when scapula is fixed) helps in elevating ribs and inhaling • When all the fibers work the muscle also creates scapular abduction from the medial line (against the antagonist rhomboid muscles) • Contraction of the inferior fibers creates external rotation of scapula and draws the inferior angle to the side and front (essential movement for raising the arm)	

Muscles affecting the shoulder girdle

Table 2.7

ORIGIN	INSERTION	ACTION	FIGURES
PECTORALIS MAJOR			
• Clavicular head: Medial 2/3 of clavicle • Sternal head: Along the external ridge of the sternum and from the cartilage of ribs 2–6 • Abdominal head: Anterior layer of the uppermost part of the rectus sheath	• Crest of greater tubercle of humerus	• Adduction and internal rotation of humerus • Horizontal adduction of arms ('hugging' movement)	
PECTORALIS MINOR			
• Connection point of cartilage of ribs 3–5	• Coracoid process of scapula	• Protraction of scapula • Depression of scapula	
TERES MINOR			
• Lateral border of scapula	• Greater tubercle of humerus	• External rotation of arm (stabilizes humerus head in shoulder joint)	
TERES MAJOR			
• Inferior dorsal 1/3 of lateral margin of scapula down to inferior angle	• Crest of lesser tubercle	• Extension, adduction and internal rotation of arm • Synergist muscle for latissimus dorsi muscle	
SUBSCAPULARIS			
• Subscapular fossa	• Lesser tubercle of humerus	• Internal rotation and adduction of arm • Stabilizes humerus head in shoulder joint	
CORACOBRACHIALIS			
• Coracoid process of scapula	• Medial surface of the humerus on the continuation of the crest of lesser tubercle	• Flexion of arm • Adduction of arm	

Kinesiological aspects

As noted, the scapula creates two synovial joints, at the connection with the clavicle (the acromioclavicular joint) and with the humerus (glenohumeral joint). In these joints, a number of movements of the scapula are possible:

- Elevation – depression
- Retraction – protraction
- External – internal rotation
- Adduction – abduction.

Scapulohumeral rhythm

An especially important movement sequence between the scapula and the humerus (the scapulohumeral rhythm) is observed mainly in movements of arm abduction–adduction.

Kinesiologically, this abduction movement can be divided into three stages (Rasch, 1989; Hamilton & Luttgens, 2002):

Stage 1: Up to about 30° in arm abduction, the scapula is fixed in place.

Stage 2: Between 30° and 90°, the scapula responds with an external rotational movement in a ratio of 2:1, that is, for every 2° of arm abduction, there is 1° of scapular rotation.

Stage 3: Beyond 90° (and up to 180°) in arm abduction, this functional ratio changes to 1:1, i.e., for every degree of arm abduction there is 1° of external rotation of the scapula.

Another aspect of upper extremity abduction is arm position in the horizontal plane. In normal situations, abduction is possible up to a range of 120°. At this point, the greater tubercle of the humerus makes contact with the acromion and is stopped. From this point, continuation of abduction of the arm up to the full range requires an external rotation of the arm that will free this mechanical "lock" (Hoppenfeld, 1976) (Fig. 2.36).

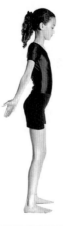

Figure 2.36 External/lateral arm rotation in order to increase range of abduction.

Normal scapulae functioning affects all the structures attached to them, creating a movement interrelationship between the arm, shoulder, chest, and spine.

An example of these movement connections can be seen in the chain reaction illustrated in Figure 2.37. Internal rotation of the arm draws the scapula into protraction and the continuation to flexion and rotation of the torso. Similarly, turning the arm outward/laterally pushes the scapula back (retraction) and causes reverse rotation of the torso. When this mechanism occurs simultaneously on both sides, the chain reaction of turning the arms inward (medially) will focus on the sagittal plane and will cause a kyphotic position of the torso.

Kinesiologically, in a condition of kyphosis of the thoracic spine, the scapulae draw forward (to a state of protraction) but as noted the effect is mutual, i.e. movement of the scapula to the rear (retraction) may affect the straightening of the torso and reduce back kyphosis (Basmajian & Slonecker, 1989) (Fig. 2.38).

To summarize this idea, it can be said that kinesiologically, the position of the scapulae affects general posture, and any reduction in their ranges of movement will harm the optimal functioning of the above-mentioned structures. For this reason, posture therapy places great emphasis on improving scapula mobility, as in many cases the postural disorder is also characterized by functional rigidity in this area.

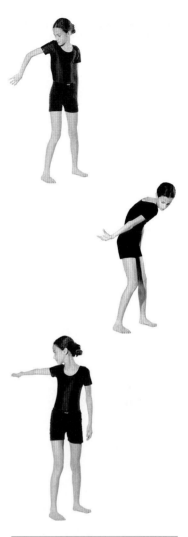

Figure 2.37 Interrelationship of the extremity joints and the torso.

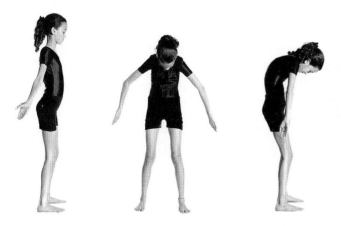

Figure 2.38 Effect of scapula position on thoracic kyphosis.

The nervous system in posture

The human nervous system enables the body to perceive feelings, to respond to changes in the environment, and to arrange and coordinate activities in its many organs and limbs. Neurophysiologists attempt to understand how the nervous system works, uncover correlations between different phenomena and find ways to intervene where biochemical and physical processes are defective or faulty. This section on the nervous system will focus mainly on functional aspects of its control over posture and movement patterns and less on anatomical aspects, namely the actual structure of the nervous system and its various elements.

As developmental processes proceed normally, maturation of the central nervous system makes precision movement function possible in the muscular system, so that work is done by the relevant muscles for a given action, while other muscles are impeded. This mechanism, which facilitates mastery of complex movements, is observable in normal coordination. Difficulty here may be evidenced by "motor overflow" or in "associated movements".

Associated movements are defined as movements that accompany a directed motor activity, but are irrelevant to the movement goal. Such movements may be found in both dynamic situations (namely faulty power regulation and difficulty in movement separation that causes energetically "uneconomical" movements) and static situations (namely excess muscle tone in various postural positions). Excess muscle tone in static situations is one of the dominant factors leading to the development of various postural disorders, because it entails an ongoing state that develops into faulty postural habits.

One of the measures of structural maturity in the central nervous system is how much myelin sheathes the nerve fibers. The myelin coating on nerve fibers permits more rapid and precise transmission of action potential; therefore, myelin sheathing level is considered a general measure of nervous system maturity (Yakovlev & Lencours, 1967). Usually most of the myelinizing process occurring after birth is completed by 2 or 3 years of age, but certain systems continue the myelinization process even in the first and second decades of life. These systems include the corpus callosum, which connects the perceptual areas between subsystems in the brain. Delayed maturation of these systems may be evidenced by coordinative difficulties and the development of postural disorders (Dennis, 1976).

When this happens, movement supervision by higher centers of the spinal cord and brain is not normal, causing processes that "stimulate" movement (motor overflow) to outnumber the processes that restrain it.

If it is assumed that the restraining mechanism in the brain cortex is responsible for control of motor overflow, it can be hypothesized that this overflow can be reduced through learning. In other words, appropriate training can significantly improve general coordination, which is a precondition for any postural improvement.

At each age, learned movement patterns reflect the interrelationships between the neural maturation process and environmental factors. In order to derive maximal benefit from constantly increasing neural ability to coordinate movement components, individuals must reduce the interference caused by faulty movement habits learned in the past. The ability to control and change faulty movement patterns learned earlier, facilitates the learning of new movement responses that "compete" with the old ones.

It is generally accepted that hereditary structures in the central nervous system determine the dominance of certain movement patterns. During maturation of the central nervous system, "inhibitive mechanisms" develop that make it possible to inhibit, overcome or assimilate these patterns (Fuchs et al., 1985). Human ability to terminate assimilated movement patterns or to inhibit them and learn new movement and postural habits depends on neural development, cognitive ability, and appropriate drilling and practice. All of these make new learning possible so that new movement patterns can be adopted more easily and rapidly.

The effect of kinesthetic ability on movement and postural patterns

One of the important functions of the nervous system in controlling movement and postural patterns is connected to the processes of receiving perceptual information. The Greek term *kinesthesia* is composed of two words: *kine* = movement, and *esthesia* = the ability to perceive or feel, that is the "perception of movement". Sherington's (1906) findings about subcutaneous and internal receptors in the human body focused on neurophysiological aspects, and the term "proprioception" often serves as a synonym for kinesthesis.

Kinesthesis as a perceptual system begins with the receptors in the muscles and joints and continues to the cerebellum and to the sensomotor areas in the cerebral cortex (Swarts, 1978; Spirduso, 1978). Some see kinesthesis as a sense through which individuals are aware of the body as a whole, of individual limbs and of the magnitude of muscle contraction.

Kinesthesis has many approaches and definitions, but what unites all those engaging in the field is the concurrence that kinesthesis is a certain type of information about movement activity and the location of body limbs. As such, kinesthetic capability is a highly important component in one's ability to maintain normal posture in static situations as well as in movement.

The main factors enabling the feeling of movement are the three types of receptors situated in the joints (joint receptors):

1. Golgi receptors – are located in the ligaments enveloping the joint and in the tendons connecting muscle to bone. These receptors provide information about the location of the joint and the direction of movement.
2. Ruffini receptors – are located inside the joint capsule in the joint itself, and mainly in the connective tissues. These receptors are highly sensitive to movement direction and speed. Ruffini receptors are affected by muscle tension, and therefore they are also active when movements are made against resistance.
3. Pacini receptors – are also located in the joint capsule, and are sensitive to rapid movements irrespective of joint direction or angle. Pacini receptors are activated by speed, acceleration and the direction of limb movement.

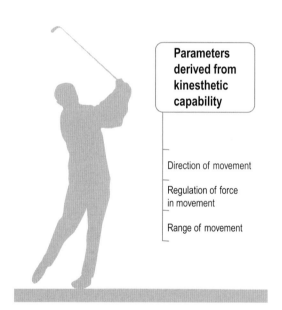

Parameters derived from kinesthetic capability

Direction of movement

Regulation of force in movement

Range of movement

Figure 2.39 Main parameters derived from kinesthetic capability.

Functioning integratively with receptors located in the muscles (muscle spindles) – the receptors described above help to maintain aligned posture and to provide information about where movement is occurring, and its range and amplitude – without any visual feedback (Fig. 2.39).

Kinesthesis is undoubtedly an important ability that affects movement and postural patterns. Body awareness, movement monitoring, learning new movements and movement memory – all these are based on kinesthetic information. This is why postural disorders will develop in most cases of kinesthetic impediments, because people have difficulty feeling the spatial placement of their body parts ("tools" for dealing with this problem in therapy will be discussed in Ch. 9).

CHAPTER 3

Postural disorders of the spine: sagittal plane

Postural disorders in the sagittal plane of the spine can be diagnosed by observation sideways and are associated with changes in the normative curvature. These conditions are characterized by larger or smaller than normal spinal curves.

Spinal curves develop gradually from one continuous arch encompassing all of the vertebrae in the embryonic stage to the curves that are characteristic of the adult human (Fig. 3.1).

Anatomically and kinesiologically, the normal range of spine curvature offers several functional advantages:

- Increased range of movement in the sagittal plane
- Shock absorption (Fig. 3.2) – the spinal curve structure helps to partially moderate the shocks

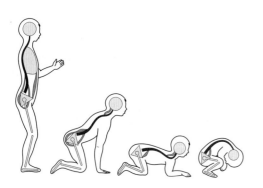

Figure 3.1 Development of spinal curves.

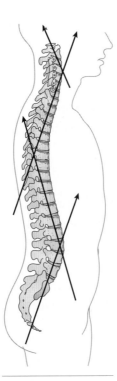

Figure 3.2 Shock absorption along the spine.

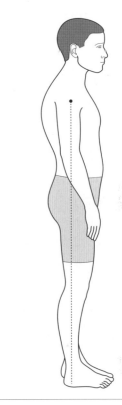

Figure 3.3 Balancing the center of gravity of the thoracic cage over the support bases.

flowing up the spine (in dynamic situations such as walking, running and jumping) so that the shocks change direction and gradually decrease in force at each curve

- Balancing the center of gravity within the support bases – the kyphotic back structure

envelops the thoracic cage and its internal organs so that the center of gravity is located above the pelvis and above the support bases on the feet (Gould & Davies, 1985). This structure helps maintain optimal posture without straining the back muscles (Fig. 3.3).

Kyphosis

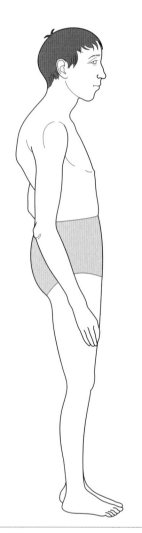

Figure 3.4 Kyphosis.

Kyphosis is the name given to a postural disorder in which the curve of the thoracic vertebrae is exaggerated and the shoulders and head assume a forward tilt (Fig. 3.4).

Other common indications of this condition are a shortening of the thoracic muscles and weakness of the upper back muscles and scapular adductors. Exaggerated curves are also likely to develop in the cervical and lumbar spine areas as compensatory processes to facilitate better body functioning. Other characteristics of this disorder are shallow breathing and low body awareness.

Functional disturbances caused by kyphosis are usually evident in several areas:

- Diminished optimal functioning of internal organs, mainly in the chest area (rigid kyphosis may damage optimal respiratory functioning)
- Difficulties in motor functioning (as a result of movement limitations)
- Tension and discomfort in the neck and shoulder girdle because of excessive muscle tone.

Possible causes of kyphosis

Kyphosis has several possible causes:

- Pathologies of the spinal vertebrae (e.g., kyphosis during adolescence caused by Scheuermann's Disease, which affects the secondary growth center of vertebral bodies)
- Imbalance between antagonist muscle groups (a combination of weakness in the upper back area and limited range of movement in the chest muscles). Muscle length is a function of the strength ratio between antagonist muscles. Imbalance between antagonist muscle groups alters the relative forces applied to specific joints and affects their alignment (Kendall & McCreary, 1983). The aim of remedial movement therapy in this case is to bring muscles to the appropriate length and strength for optimal posture and functioning
- Psychological factors, such as emotional stress and low self esteem, among adolescent females for example. Here the tendency is towards "rounding the shoulders", as though the growing girl is trying to "hide" her developing breasts. This usually occurs when the adolescent is ashamed of the natural processes she is undergoing and tries to hide them
- Low body awareness and faulty movement habits in daily activities. Deficient movement patterns have a negative effect on the musculoskeletal system and in time, cumulative damage can lead to postural disorders.

Main areas of treatment of kyphosis *(Fig. 3.5)*

- Exercises to maintain normal pelvic position – to create a basis for correct alignment of the spine.

  According to the kinematic chain principle, pelvic position and stability directly affect spinal alignment. The main factors involved in pelvic stabilization are muscles and ligaments. Balance depends on equilibrium between antagonist muscle groups responsible for movement on the sagittal plane in anterior and posterior pelvic tilt.

- Exercises to stretch and lengthen the chest muscles (pectoralis major/pectoralis minor)

  The chest muscles are essential for good range of movement of the shoulder girdle, and shortened chest muscles will affect the alignment of the entire torso. Lengthening these muscles reduces their resistance to the back muscles (antagonists) and thus allows the scapulae to remain in their proper position without being drawn forward.

- Strengthening the upper back muscles, the deep erector spinae and the shoulder extensors (principles for balanced strengthening of the back muscles appear in Chapter 8).

- Breathing exercises for increasing range of respiration (especially inhalation).

  In general, breathing depends on the joints connected to the thoracic area. Good movement of these joints facilitates full, free breathing, while constraints on some or all of them will adversely affect respiratory processes.

- In addition to the chest muscles mentioned above, movement of the joints connecting thorax and ribs (the sterno-costal joints) and those linking ribs and vertebrae (the costo-vertebral joints) is of great importance for maintaining chest flexibility and optimal respiratory functioning (Kisner & Colby, 1985).

- Aerobic activity for improving cardiopulmonary endurance (such as running, long-distance walking, swimming and bicycle riding).

- Mobility exercises for the thoracic vertebrae (T1–12) on all movement planes, from a variety of starting positions.

  This is extremely important especially in treating structural kyphosis, which is characterized by rigidity and functional stiffness of the thoracic vertebrae.

- Exercises to increase hamstring flexibility and thus improve functional pelvic mobility on the sagittal plane (in anterior and posterior pelvic tilt).

- Awareness and relaxation exercises.

In addition to strength and flexibility exercises, it is recommended that patients be taught correct muscle activation (posture awareness), for example, how to use the abdominal muscles correctly in exercises performed while standing, better control of anterior and posterior pelvic tilt mobility, and developing kinesthetic capabilities with eyes open and closed.

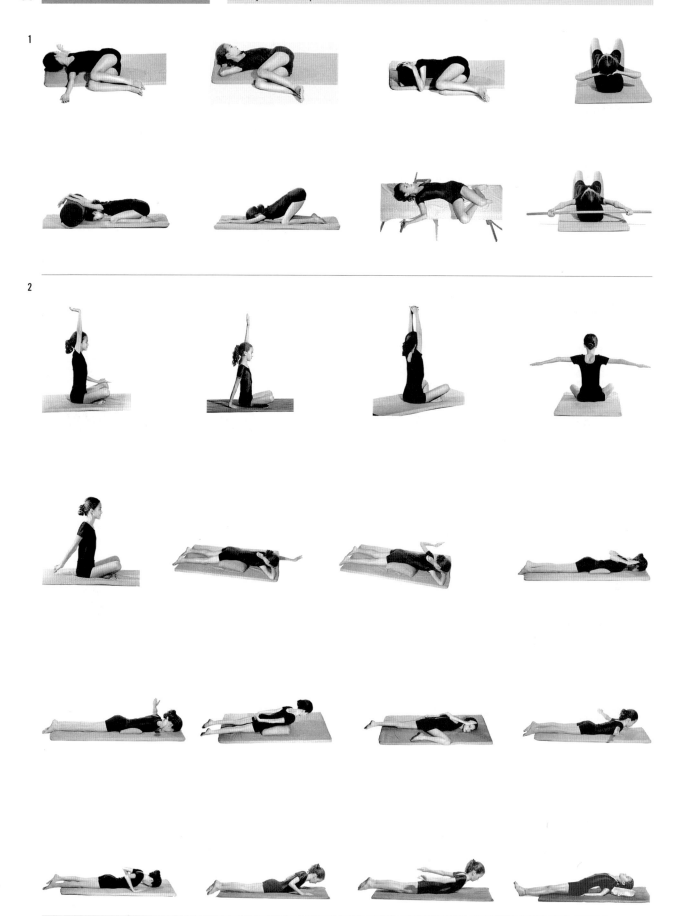

Figure 3.5 Examples of exercises suitable for treating kyphosis. (For a detailed description of these exercises, see Ch. 8.)

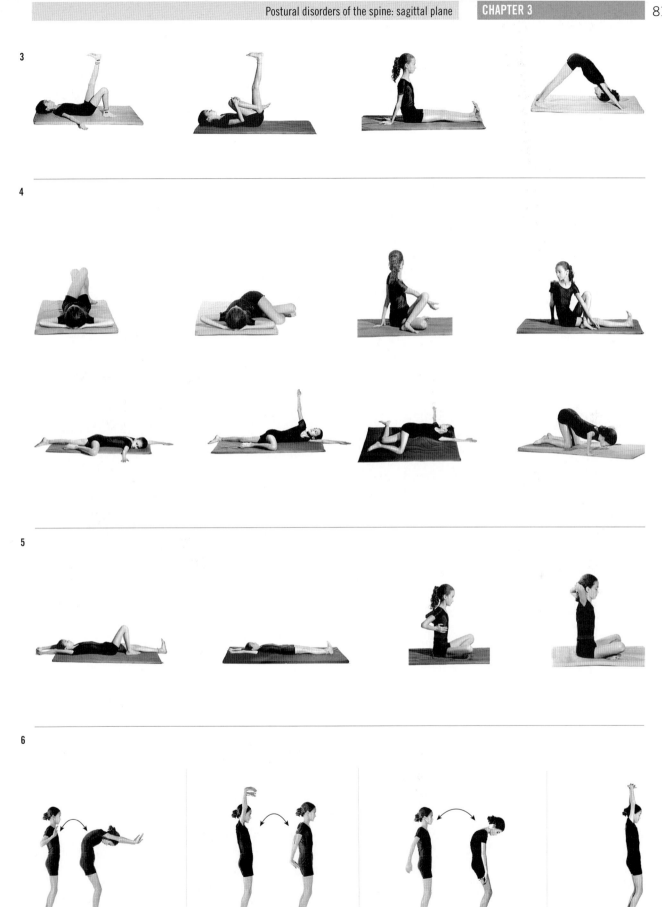

Figure 3.5 (*continued*).

Lordosis

Lordosis is a state of exaggerated curvature of the lumbar spine with excessive anterior pelvic tilt (Fig. 3.6A). In this condition, body weight is transferred from the strong, broad, supportive portion of the vertebral bodies to the more delicate arches, and at the same time, the spinous processes move closer than usual to one another (Fig. 3.6B). This narrows the vertebral foramina through which the nerves pass, a process which over time may generate pressure on nerve roots in the lumbar area (Cyriax, 1979; Waddel, 1996).

Characteristic signs of lordosis

- Exaggerated lumbo-pelvic angle – more than 60° in women and 55° in men. (An explanation of pelvic angle appears in Ch. 2, Fig. 2.19)
- Protruding concavity of the lumbar vertebrae
- Protruding and slack belly
- Protruding buttocks
- Hyperextension of the knees (genu-recurvatum) (characteristic of hyper-flexibility)
- Flat feet.

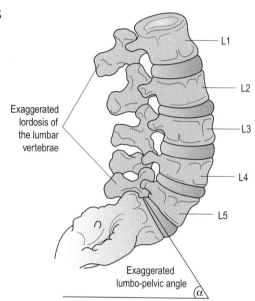

Figure 3.6B Skeletal lordosis.

Possible causes of lordosis

- Shortening of the muscles that tilt the pelvis anteriorly
- Weakness of the muscles that tilt the pelvis posteriorly
- Structural changes in the vertebrae
- Shortening of the ligaments and the fascia covering the posterior surface of the waist
- Faulty movement habits
- Hereditary structure
- Unbalanced alignment of joints in the lower extremities (ankle, knee, hip)
- Injury to the lumbar vertebrae. Examples of structural injuries that could cause lordosis are sacralization of vertebra L5 or spondylolisthesis – a state characterized by forward movement of a vertebra in relation to the one below it.

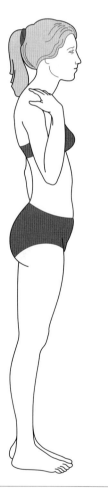

Figure 3.6A Lordosis.

Lordosis is a postural disorder that can appear in two forms

1. Flexible lordosis – which can be corrected by conscious effort.

   Possible characteristics of this form are weakness of the muscles that create posterior pelvic tilt (abdominals, gluteus maximus, semitendinosus, semimembranosus, and biceps femoris).

2. Structural lordosis – which cannot be corrected by conscious effort.

   Possible characteristics of this form are shortening of the erector spinae muscles in the lumbar region and shortening of the muscles that create anterior pelvic tilt (the iliopsoas, which in this state pulls the lumbar vertebrae forward, the rectus femoris, the quadratus lumborum and the sartorius) (Fig. 3.7).

Main areas of treatment of lordosis *(Fig. 3.8)*

- Lengthening the muscles that create anterior pelvic tilt and making them more flexible
- Strengthening and shortening the muscles that create posterior pelvic tilt

  The abdominal muscle group plays an important role in posterior pelvic tilt. Weakness in these muscles may cause excessive anterior tilt and thus (in a chain reaction) affect stability of the lower back (abdominal weakness, damage to pelvic stability, anterior pelvic tilt and increasing lumbar lordosis)

- Learning to control normal pelvic position

  Kinesiologically, the position of the pelvis affects the alignment of the lumbar vertebrae above it. If the pelvis is balanced, the vertebrae above it will also be in balance. But a pelvis tilted forward adversely affects the lumbar vertebral position, causing excessive lumbar lordosis (the chain principle) (Gould & Davies, 1985; Norkin & Levangie, 1993)

  It is important to exercise the muscles that stabilize the pelvis. Muscles are the key to altering and controlling this disorder, since they respond to the environment and are controlled by conscious thinking processes. Nevertheless, the complex functioning of the muscles encircling the pelvis makes it difficult for many patients to comprehend, internalize and produce correct pelvic position. The way to address this problem is through clear guidance and extensive drills for improving mastery of anterior and posterior pelvic movements. Drills of this type will contribute to an understanding of the functional links between pelvic position and spinal curves

- Learning proper use of the whole spine – and especially the lower back

  Kinesiologically, the lumbar region is designed for both mobility and weight-bearing. But despite their good structural design for both tasks, lumbar vertebrae cannot both move and bear weight at the same time. These contradictory skills are the main reason for lumbar vertebral vulnerability to injury.

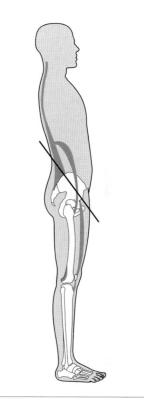

Figure 3.7 Muscles creating anterior pelvic tilt.

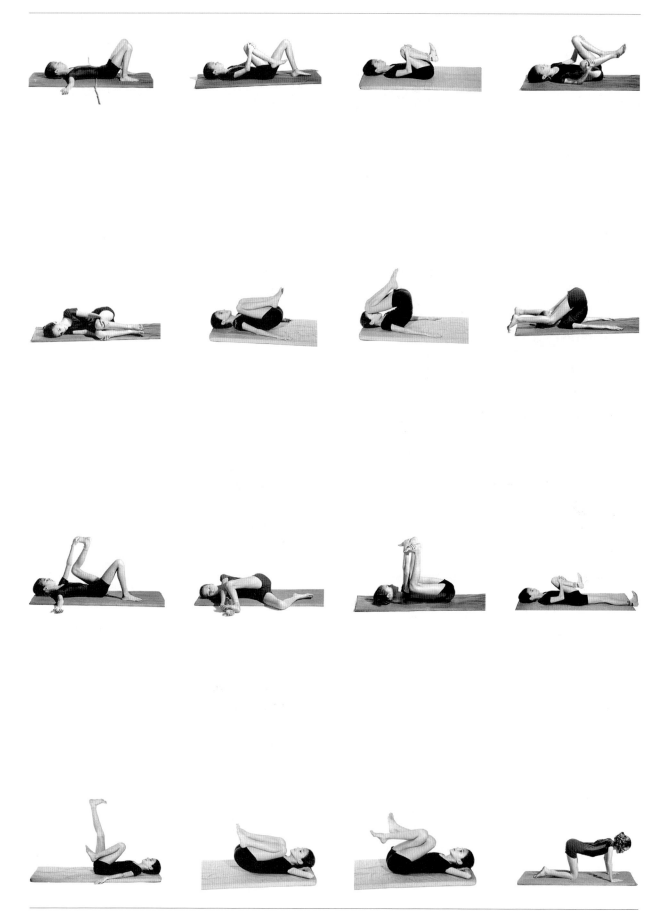

Figure 3.8 Examples of exercises and starting positions suitable for treating lordosis. (For a more detailed description of these exercises, see Ch. 8.)

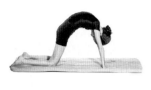
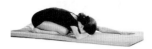
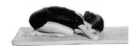
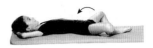

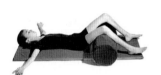
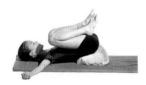
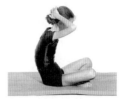

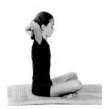
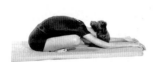
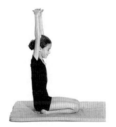

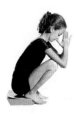
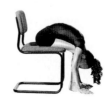
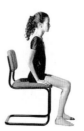

Figure 3.8 (*continued*).

Flat back

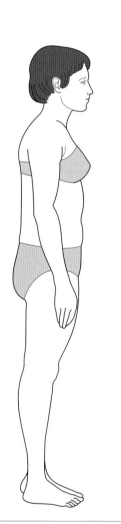

Figure 3.9 Flat back.

This disorder, with relation to the norm, is characterized by decreased lumbar lordosis (Fig. 3.9). Aside from genetics, other reasons for its development include weakness of hip flexors and short hamstrings, which together influence the position of the pelvis and create posterior pelvic tilt.

In many cases, flat back is also accompanied by serious low back pain symptoms, traceable to the intervertebral discs in the lumbar spine. Because it is intended to facilitate movement and absorb shocks, the structure of the disc is also sensitive to pressure and to shear forces working on it (Cyriax, 1979).

The anatomical structure of the spine is characterized by curvatures that need to be maintained within normal ranges. Lordosis in the cervical and lumbar areas creates a wider gap on the anterior side of the vertebrae and a narrower gap on their posterior side (Fig. 3.10). As a result, regular light forward-directed pressure is maintained on the intervertebral disc as it bears weight. When the spinal column is flexed, disc pressure is directed to the posterior, creating pressure on the dura in the spinal canal through the posterior longitudinal ligament. In some cases, this pressure may cause pain.

Cervical and lumbar lordoses play an important role in protecting the posterior longitudinal ligament from excessive strain and reducing pressure on the anterior side of the vertebral joints (Cyriax, 1979). Obviously, then, when vertebrae lie flat on one another (as in flat back), less forward flexion of the spine is required to create pressure on the posterior section of the disc (Fig. 3.11). In normal posture, the lordosis directs pressure towards the spinal canal only in cases of considerable forward flexion of the spinal column.

This explains the importance of lumbar lordosis in raising the threshold for posterior intervertebral pressure during flexion (Fig. 3.10). This important 'safety mechanism' is missing in flat back, which is why back pain is so common among people with this disorder. Thus, flat back can be defined as a complex disorder involving functional disturbances of both the musculoskeletal system and the nervous system.

Main areas of exercise for flat back *(Fig. 3.12)*

- Exercise to maintain normal pelvic position – for optimal alignment of the spine and for encouraging anterior pelvic tilt on the sagittal plane
- Hamstring flexibility and lengthening exercises, to improve anterior pelvic tilt
- Strengthening hip flexors
- Exercise to improve general lower back vertebral mobility.

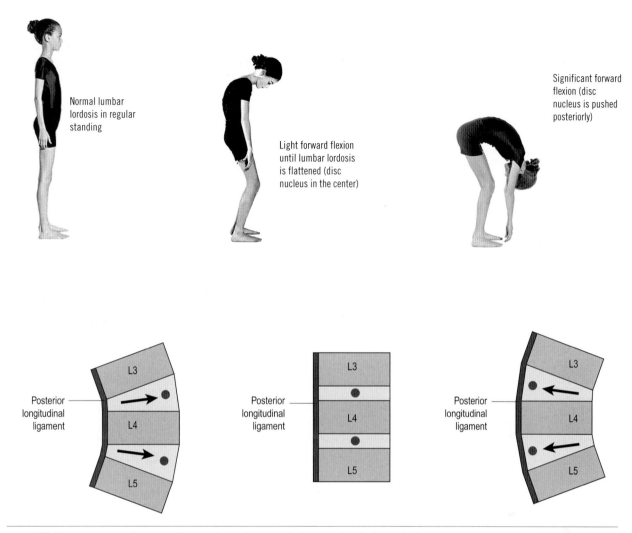

Figure 3.10 State of the intervertebral discs of the lower back vertebrae and the lumbar lordosis "safety mechanism".

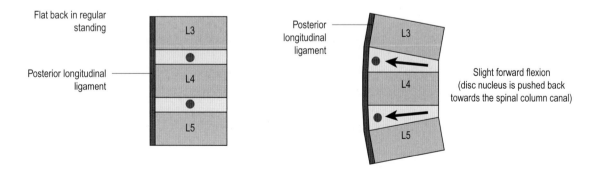

Figure 3.11 Intervertebral discs in flat back.

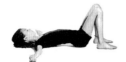
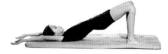

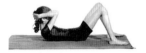
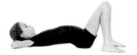
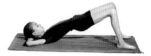

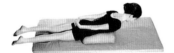
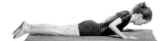
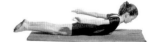

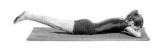
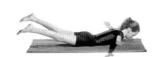
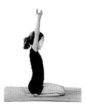

Figure 3.12 Examples of exercises and starting positions for treating flat back. (For a more detailed description of these exercises, see Ch. 8.)

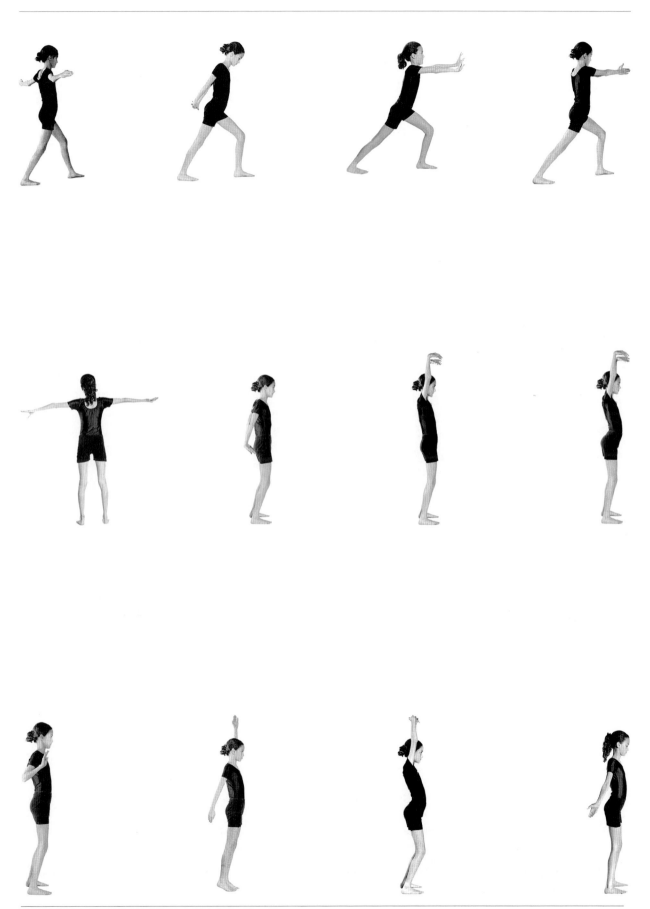

Figure 3.12 (*continued*).

Injuries to the intervertebral disc

The intervertebral disc is composed of a sheath of stratified ligaments (the anulus fibrosus) that encapsulates a gel-like substance known as the nucleus pulposus (Fig. 3.13). The discs separating the vertebrae serve as spinal column shock absorbers. They "give" in response to the pressure of weights activated upon them and then return to their original shape when the weight is removed. The special structure of the disc creates a kind of hydraulic system in which the soft inner part distributes pressure equally in all directions throughout the length of the spinal column (Cyriax, 1979).

Under normal conditions, without pressures and weights, the circular anulus fibrosus enveloping the gelatinous nucleus of the disc is strong enough to support the nucleus and keep it centered between the vertebral bodies. However, prolonged exposure to loads on the spinal column may result in injury to the disc (Nachemson, 1983) in one of two common forms:

1. *Protrusion*: This is a case in which a small tear occurs in the anulus fibrosus, weakening support for the nucleus pulposus. If this occurs, not all of the gel flows into the spinal column canal, and the pressure exerted on the spinal cord or on the nerve root is very light. If any damage to the intervertebral disc is diagnosed, therapeutic exercise should be applied only under medical supervision. As the type of activity should be adapted specifically to the type of problem, an unprofessional approach may be dangerous and may aggravate the condition (Fig. 3.14).

2. *Disc herniation*: This is a case of severe damage to the disc, with a partial seepage of the nucleus pulposus outside the disc boundaries and resultant pressure on the neural structures (Fig. 3.15).

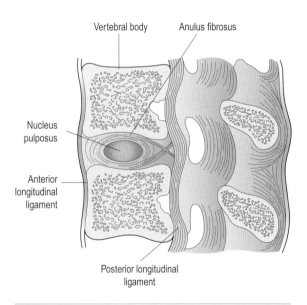

Figure 3.13 The intervertebral disc. If any damage to the intervertebral disc is diagnosed, therapeutic exercise should be applied only under medical supervision. As the type of activity should be adapted specifically to the type of problem, an unprofessional approach may be dangerous and may aggravate the condition.

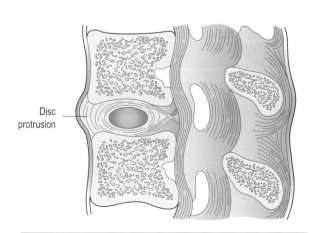

Figure 3.14 Disc protrusion.

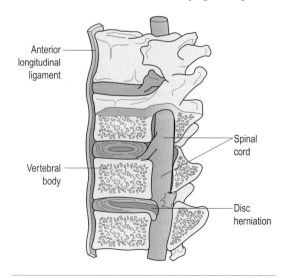

Figure 3.15 Disc herniation.

Relaxed posture

Relaxed posture is characterized by forward movement of the pelvis, slouched shoulders, and possibly a flattening of the lumbar curve with increased thoracic curve (Fig. 3.16). This is a disorder characterized in many cases by low body awareness and faulty movement patterns.

The development of relaxed posture may be attributable to any number of factors, among them general weakness, fatigue and faulty movement habits, combined with emotional difficulties such as low self-esteem and lack of self-confidence.

The main problem of relaxed posture is that malfunctioning of a weak muscular system overloads the supportive ligament system. The result is a "vicious cycle" that adversely affects general posture among those with relaxed posture (Fig. 3.17).

Main areas of exercise for relaxed posture *(Fig. 3.18)*

- Strengthening upper back muscles and shoulder girdle
- Strengthening abdominal muscles
- Strengthening leg muscles
- Extensive work on body awareness for improving body alignment and postural patterns (also see Ch. 9).

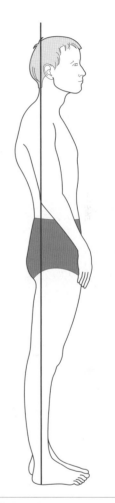

Figure 3.16 Relaxed posture.

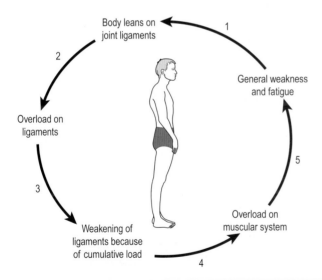

Figure 3.17 The common mechanism for developing relaxed posture.

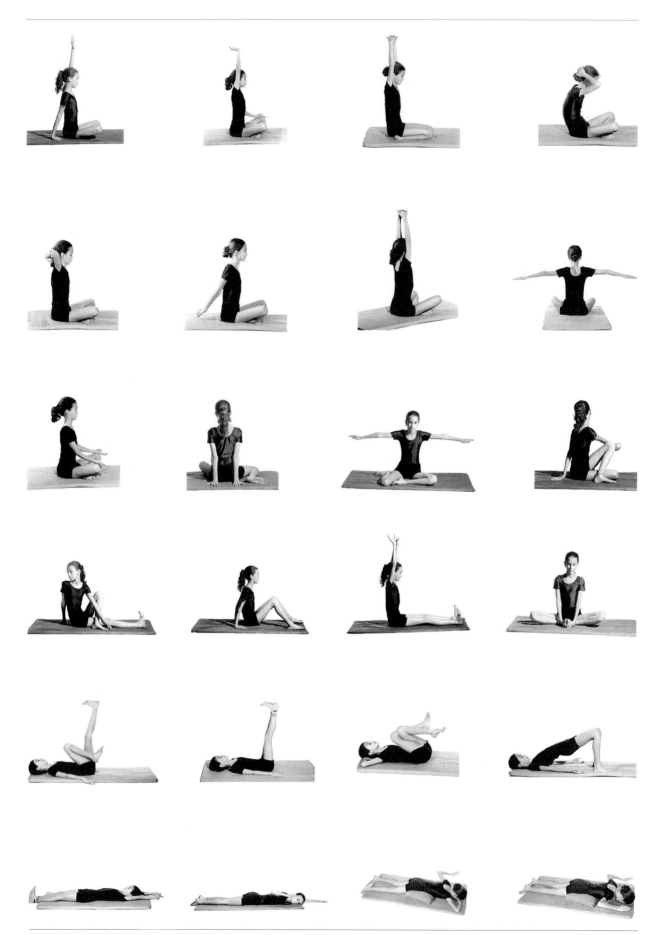

Figure 3.18 Examples of exercises suitable for the treatment of relaxed posture. (For a more detailed description of these exercises, see Ch.8.)

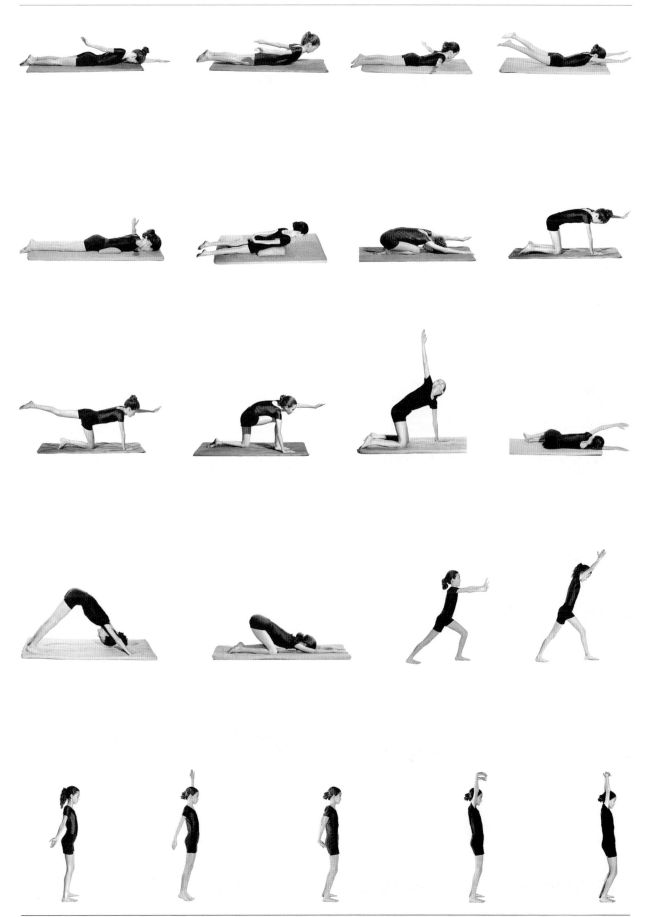

Figure 3.18 (*continued*).

CHAPTER 4

Postural disorders of the spine: coronal/ frontal plane

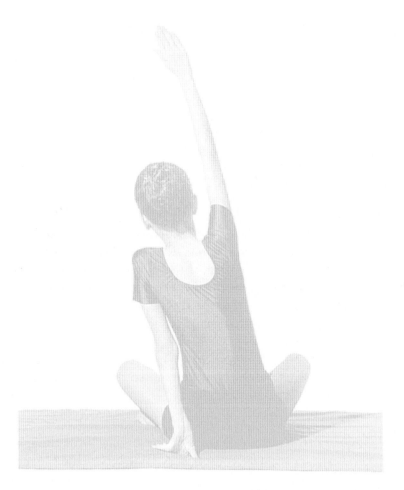

Postural disorders in the coronal/frontal plane of the spinal column can be diagnosed through observation from the back or the front, and are observable as an imbalance in the spinal column and on both sides of the torso.

Many variations of spinal-column deviation from the median line are defined as scoliosis. This chapter surveys these complex disorders and discusses ways of diagnosing and of treating them through movement. Scoliosis is a lateral deviation of the spinal column from the median, usually accompanied by rotation of the vertebrae. Scoliosis can take many forms, in terms of angle of deviation and of indications and symptoms, therefore familiarity with its many associated parameters is necessary for proper understanding of the disorder.

Parameters used in determining scoliosis

- Direction (to the right, the left or several directions)
- Location (boundaries of the deviation in terms of affected vertebrae)
- Angle
- Structural imbalance in terms of anthropometric parameters (such as different lengths of the lower extremities)
- Functional imbalance (such as overt differences in muscle tone and in range of motion between the two sides of the body)
- Secondary visual indications (such as asymmetric fat folds on either side of the body)
- Functional motor difficulties (for example, in static and dynamic balance)
- Classification as either structural scoliosis or functional scoliosis.

The following pages describe the most common characteristics of each parameter.

Direction of scoliosis

Scoliosis may take on one of two possible shapes:

1. *"C" shape*: C-shaped scoliosis is characterized by a curvature of the spinal column to one side. The deviation may be centered in one area of the spine (such as the thoracic vertebrae) or it may also include the lumbar vertebrae. The designation of the "C" disorder as right or left always refers to the side of the curvature, that is, if the right side is curved, the scoliosis is defined as "C" to the right and vice versa (Fig. 4.1).

    As the disorder is characterized by visible imbalance along the length of the body, certain typical indications should be recognized:

- Unequal shoulder height: the shoulder on the side with the curvature is higher
- Unequal distance of the scapulae from the spinal column: the scapula on the concave side is closer to the median
- The inferior angle of the scapula on the concave side is lower
- Distortion of the rib cage, which can take several shapes, such as rib hump in cases of rotation in the thoracic vertebrae
- Imbalance in ilium bone height: the ilium ridge on the concave side is higher
- Unequal distance of arms from the torso: the arm on the curved side seems closer to the torso
- Unequal fat folds in the lumbar and cervical areas: fat folds may appear on the concave side.

*These external indications of the C-shape disorder are highly generalized. Each case should be examined individually because this type of scoliosis can assume any number of variations, and not all the above-mentioned symptoms will necessarily appear.

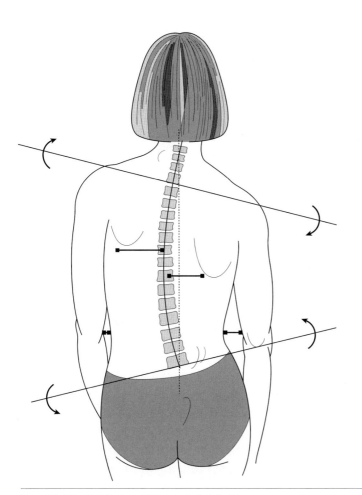

Figure 4.1 Characteristic signs of C-type scoliosis to the left.

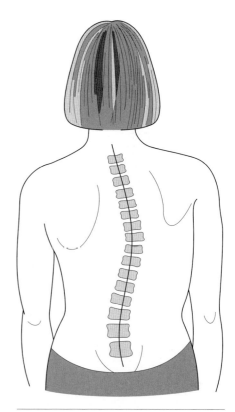

Figure 4.2 S-type scoliosis (right thoracic, left lumbar).

2. *"S" shape*: S-shaped scoliosis is characterized by at least two curves with deviations from both sides of the median line of the spinal column, for example, a superior curvature to the right in the thoracic area, and an inferior curvature to the left in the lumbar area. In this case, the definition of the disorder pertains to the sides of the spinal column that are curved (Figs 4.2, 4.3).

   S-shaped scoliosis usually involves one primary curvature and one additional secondary (compensatory) curvature. Because deviation directions are not uniform, treatment in this type of disorder is more complex and requires extra caution.

Scoliosis location

The boundaries of scoliosis are determined by the vertebrae that deviate laterally from the median. The disorder may be concentrated in one specific area of the cervical spine (cervical scoliosis), the thoracic spine (thoracic scoliosis) or in the lumbar area (lumbar scoliosis), or it may implicate many vertebrae in several regions and in different variations. Precise delineation regarding the boundaries of the scoliosis is possible only by means of X-ray.

Scoliosis angle

Scoliosis angle, which is measured on the X-ray, is important in determining the severity of the disorder. The larger the scoliosis angle, the more severe the disorder is. Scoliosis angle is important both for diagnostic purposes and for monitoring progression of the disorder. The technique for measuring the angle will be presented later in this chapter (see Figs 4.14, 4.15).

Rotation in the spinal vertebrae

Rotation in the spinal vertebrae indicates a significant degree of scoliosis. Usually, rotation occurs in the thoracic vertebrae, and is denoted by a protuberance of the ribs on one side of the upper back when bending forward (Fig 4.4, and see Fig. 4.7). Some cases of flexible functional scoliosis show no evidence of vertebral rotation, and therefore an examination to determine whether such rotation exists is an important part of the diagnosis.

Structural imbalance in terms of anthropometric parameters

Scoliosis may sometimes develop from an imbalance originating in the skeletal system. Differences in the length of the lower limbs, for example, may create an imbalance in pelvic position, which will later appear as a disorder in the alignment of the spinal column caused by an out-of-balance base. Scoliosis of this type requires different treatment and cannot be resolved by therapeutic exercise only. The anthropometric examinations discussed later in this chapter are an important component of the diagnostic process because they may provide clues as to the source of the disorder.

Functional imbalance in the musculoskeletal system

Scoliosis is also usually characterized by obvious functional differences on either side of the body. This imbalance may be measurable in terms of ranges of motion or muscle strength, and is usually discernible in the shoulder girdle, back, and spinal column mobility, and movement in the lower extremities.

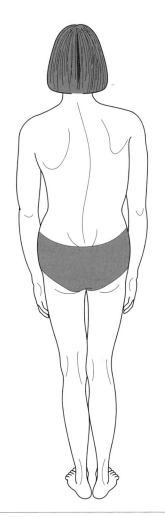

Figure 4.3 Characteristic signs of S-type scoliosis.

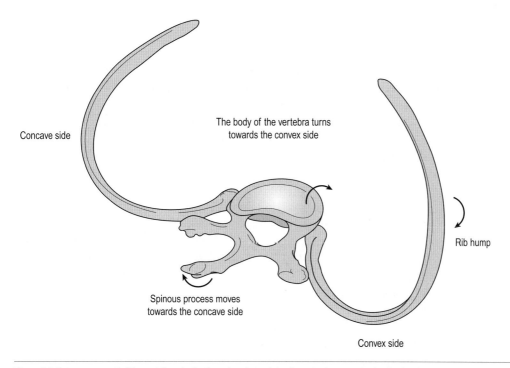

Figure 4.4 Rotary movement of the vertebrae in the thoracic spine and the distortion it creates in the ribs (posterior view).

Secondary visual indications

The most typical visual indications of scoliosis are illustrated in Figures 4.1 and 4.3. It is important to remember that the presence of specific markers does not necessarily indicate that real scoliosis exists in the spinal column. In other words, *the diagnosis of scoliosis cannot be based solely on external indications*. The final diagnosis of scoliosis always entails X-rays as well.

Functional motor difficulties

Normal development enables children to attain functional independence while posturally erect and to withstand the forces of gravity while sitting, walking, running, climbing, etc. They learn to adapt their senso-motoric function to changing demands during daily activities.

In certain cases, the characteristic imbalance of scoliosis may impair normal motor functioning, mainly in the following areas

- Coordination:
  Good coordination creates a dynamic posture that facilitates both adjustment of movement to the stabilizing areas and movement that adapts itself to changing needs in daily activities (Ratzon, 1993). It should be remembered that an important prerequisite for developing efficient, harmonious and coordinated mobility is an integration of

posture and mobility: the body must be sufficiently balanced and stable to allow efficient movement functioning.

- Balance:
  Difficulties here are evident in both static and dynamic balance, and are linked to the ability to freely shift the base of support in a manner that creates a flowing, smooth transition from one position to another (Geissele et al., 1991).

- Vertical organization of the body due to kinesthetic problems:
  In many cases, prolonged scoliosis may impair body image and kinesthesis. This is evident in individuals who have difficulty "finding" their midline and organizing and balancing their limbs around it. One indication of such a situation is the feeling that one's body is "twisted" when in fact it is balanced. This aspect of kinesthetic work is a very important element in movement treatment for scoliosis.

Classifying scoliosis as structural or functional

Scoliosis can develop in a variety of forms, but most types can be classified as either:

1. Functional scoliosis (flexible) or
2. Structural scoliosis (rigid).

Functional scoliosis (flexible)

Flexible or functional scoliosis refers to a disorder in which there are no structural changes in the skeletal system (spinal vertebrae) or pathology in ligaments and muscles.

Several criteria usually indicate that scoliosis is flexible

- When lying on the back, the scoliosis disappears
- In forward bending, the scoliosis disappears
- A person who is aware of the scoliosis can correct it volitionally.

Possible causes of flexible functional scoliosis

- Incorrect movement patterns that entail asymmetric use of the body in daily activities (such as carrying objects, prolonged sitting, prolonged reading in an asymmetric position, lack of physical awareness, etc.)
- Imbalance in antagonistic muscle group strength on either side of the spinal column. This imbalance may also be the product of occupational activities, intense-training sports, unbalanced physical training, etc.
- Differences in the length of the lower limbs caused by pathological factors (accidents, fractures, postural disorders in the ankle or knee position, etc.), or developmental factors (a transient stage in the child's growth processes). In each of these situations, shoe inserts to balance leg length may balance the pelvis and solve the problem.

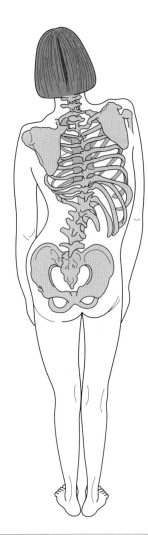

Figure 4.5 Structural scoliosis.

Structural scoliosis (rigid)

Structural (rigid) scoliosis refers to a disorder involving physical changes in the structure of the skeletal system (spinal vertebrae) (Fig. 4.5). In many cases, untreated flexible scoliosis may evolve into a rigid disorder at a higher level of severity.

The following criteria usually indicate structural scoliosis

- Rotation in thoracic vertebrae. Such rotation causes asymmetry in the ribs of the thoracic cage and a considerable protuberance of one side of the upper back (rib hump). This protrusion is especially evident while bending forward, and usually appears on the convex side of the spinal column
- Spinal column deviation from the midline cannot be corrected independently by the patient, and causes functional imbalance in other parts of the body such as the shoulder girdle, lower back or hips.

Possible causes of structural scoliosis This disorder appears in a number of forms, at different ages and for diverse reasons (some of them genetic) that cannot always be clearly diagnosed. Therefore, most cases of structural scoliosis are described in orthopedic medicine as "idiopathic scoliosis", that is, scoliosis of unknown cause. At the same time, many studies dealing with the etiology of the disorder offer a broad range of suppositions and theories as to possible reasons for scoliosis:

- Imbalance in the antagonistic muscles located on either side of the spinal column (Alter, 1988; Nudelman & Reis, 1990) (Fig. 4.6) – asymmetry in muscle tone can be caused by any number of factors such as improper movement habits over time, accident-engendered injury to muscles on one side, neurological problems, disease, surgery, etc.
- Asymmetry in pelvic position (Wagner, 1990) – such asymmetry may be the result of any number of factors, such as differences in the lower limb length, improper positioning of the hip joint on one side, faulty positioning of the foot and ankle, etc.
- Asymmetrical growth of the thoracic cage or of spinal vertebrae as a result of developmental deficiencies (such as hemivertebra) (Roaf, 1978; Brown, 1988; Stokes & Gardner, 1991)
- Rapid and unbalanced growth of the skeletal system during adolescence (Loncar et al., 1991)
- Hormonal control deficiencies affecting control over spinal column growth, mainly among adolescent girls (Nicolopoulus et al., 1985).

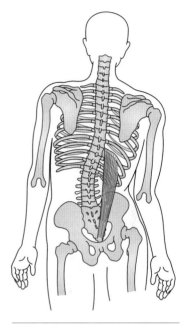

Figure 4.6 Imbalance in antagonistic muscle groups (Nudelman & Reis, 1990).

Diagnosing scoliosis

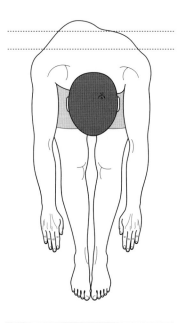

Figure 4.7 Rib hump examination: Examining upper back balance in forward bending.

Of the many postural disorders commonly found in the population, scoliosis is the most complex and the most difficult to diagnose and treat. Proper diagnosis is extremely important for designing a coordinated exercise program and reliably monitoring progress during treatment (Solberg, 1996a).

To diagnose scoliosis, special tests must be used in addition to the standard posture tests detailed in Chapter 7. They include the following stages:

1. Subjective evaluation of patient in a standing position.
   Physical asymmetry is examined in the following areas:

   • Shoulder height
   • Scapular position
   • Chest area, pelvic and hip joint position
   • Lateral deviation of the spinal column (clinical evidence of scoliosis).

2. Examination of vertebral rotation (rib hump) (Fig. 4.7).
   Standing: Bending torso forward, legs together, knees extended and shoulders relaxed.
   Practitioner makes a subjective evaluation of imbalance or protuberance (hump) in the upper back area.

3. Objective measurements (Solberg, 1994).

   a. Demographic data, such as child's age, weight, height and other cases of scoliosis in the family. It is also recommended to obtain information about the child's motor development and medical history.

   b. Anthropometric tests: These tests are intended to gather information about lateral asymmetry throughout the body and include the following measurements (Solberg, 1996b):

   • *Height of acromia*: the vertical distance between each scapula (acromion) to the floor
   • *Scapula–spine distance*: measured horizontally from the inferior angle of each scapula to the nearest thoracic vertebral spinous process (Fig. 4.8)
   • *S1–acromia distance*: the distance between the apex of the right and left scapulae (acromia) to vertebra S1 (both in standing and forward bending positions) (Fig. 4.9)
   • *Biacromial diameter*: maximum distance between right and left acromia. The measurement is taken from behind using an anthropometer (patient is standing)

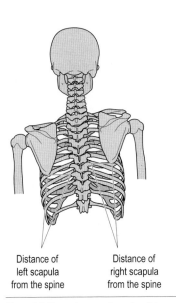

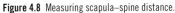

Distance of
left scapula
from the spine

Distance of
right scapula
from the spine

Figure 4.8 Measuring scapula–spine distance.

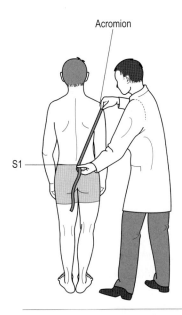

Acromion

S1

Figure 4.9 Measuring the distance between right and left acromia to vertebra S1 (should be measured in both standing and bending positions).

- *Asymmetry in the shoulder girdle* (Solberg 1994, 1996a): this objective test examines the asymmetry angle of the scapulae (α), utilizing data obtained by measuring biacromial diameter (o) and measuring height differences between the acromia (h), as shown in Figure 4.10. Thus, the angle of deviation is calculated as follows:

$$h/o \; Arc \; Sin = \alpha$$

- *Height of the anterior superior iliac spine* (ASIS): vertical distance from both sides of the pelvis to the floor

- *Lower limb length*: measured from the anterior superior iliac spine (ASIS) to the medial malleolus of the ankle (with the subject lying supine) (Fig. 4.11).

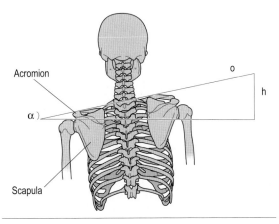

Acromion

α)

Scapula

o

h

Figure 4.10 Measuring scapulae angle of deviation: = h/o Arc Sin.

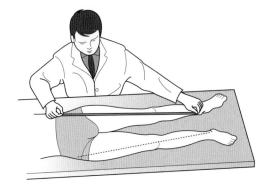

Figure 4.11 Measuring lower limb length.

4. Functional tests.

The functional tests are intended to help diagnosticians locate functional imbalances in the body, and mainly to identify significant differences in ranges of motion between the two sides of the body.

a. Lateral bending (patient is seated) – measurement of the distance between C7 to the sitting surface while patient bends to the right and to the left (Fig. 4.12A,B). It is recommended that another person or support bands be used to stabilize the pelvis, as illustrated in Figure 4.12A.

b. Shoulder girdle flexibility (patient is seated) – this test provides a general picture of range of motion in the shoulder girdle. Patients raise one elbow and try to touch the area between their scapulae with their hand. The second hand is placed on the lower back, hand facing out, and patients try to elevate their lower hand and try to reach the fingers of the upper hand. Using a ruler, measurement is made of the distance between the hands (if they do not touch) or the finger overlap (if they do) for both sides (Fig. 4.13).

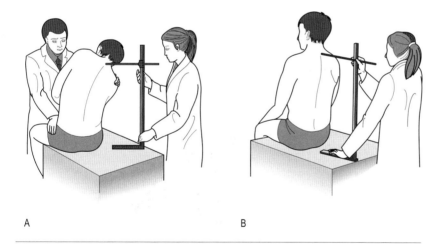

A   B

Figure 4.12 (A,B) Measuring differences in range of motion during lateral bending of spine.

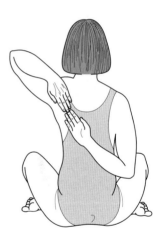

Figure 4.13 General flexibility of the shoulder girdle.

5. X-rays (COBB angle).

It is common practice to measure the angle of scoliosis on an X-ray (Fig. 4.14). Measuring the angle of scoliosis includes the following steps (Fig. 4.15):

a. Defining the boundaries of scoliosis – a line is drawn parallel to the upper part of the vertebra with the greatest deviation (line A in Fig. 4.15).

b. Similarly, another line is then drawn parallel to the vertebra located at the lower boundary of the scoliosis (line B in Fig. 4.15).

c. A vertical line is drawn from each of these lines.

The angle that is formed at the meeting of these lines – defined as the "angle of scoliosis" represents the degree of severity of scoliosis (angle "α" in Fig. 4.15).

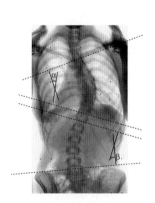

Figure 4.14 Measuring the angle of scoliosis on an X-ray (COBB angle).

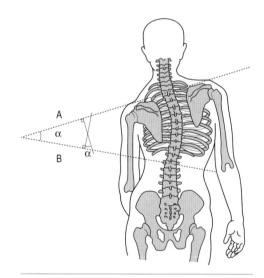

Figure 4.15 Measuring the COBB angle.

Therapeutic exercise for scoliosis

Treating scoliosis through remedial exercise is a controversial issue. Many studies of the effect of therapeutic exercise on scoliosis have found that the disorder continues to progress despite the exercise. These results cast doubt on the effectiveness of movement exercise for improving spinal alignment (Roaf, 1978; Stone et al., 1979; Keim, 1982; Kisner & Colby, 1985).

In 1941, the American Orthopedic Association came to the conclusion that the use of exercises should be avoided in treating scoliosis. This conclusion was based on a study of 435 patients of whom 60% manifested a worsening of the angle of scoliosis and the remaining 40% registered no change. Stone et al. (1979) examined the effect of remedial exercise on 99 patients during a 9-month period and reported similar results.

However, closer examination of these studies reveals some important flaws:

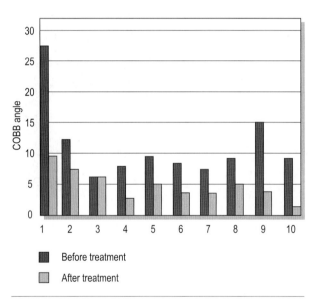

Figure 4.16 The effect of therapeutic exercise on the angle of scoliosis (Solberg, 1996a).

- Most of the studies dealt with large populations. Using remedial exercise for treating scoliosis requires a limited number of patients because of the complexity of the disorder. As the number of participants increases, treatment effectiveness and quality decline
- The exercise "treatment" consisted of a few exercises that the children learned in one or two meetings. These exercises were performed by the children independently at home for a few months
- In all the studies reviewed, there was inadequate monitoring of the quality and frequency of the children's exercise performance; in other words, no one checked whether the children actually followed instructions pertaining to how and how often to perform the exercises
- Examinations at the end of the research period revealed that a significant percentage of the children had forgotten part of the exercises or had been performing them incorrectly.

Clearly, therefore, without close supervision and constant monitoring of performance quality, any information about the effect of therapeutic exercises on scoliosis is unreliable and cannot be used for drawing clear conclusions about the effectiveness of such treatment.

In a study conducted by this author, the problems detracting from reliability of the previous studies were taken into account and changes were introduced in the research design to ensure constant monitoring of performance of the therapeutic exercises (Solberg, 1996a). The main changes in the study were as follows:

- The research population was small, permitting personalized quality treatment on a three-meetings-per-week basis
- Each child was given exercises especially and precisely adapted to his/her physical status, based on the diagnostic results obtained. This aspect is critically important because of the large number of parameters delineating individual cases of scoliosis, including deviation angle, direction and location, patient's age, gender and physique, and type of scoliosis (structural or functional)
- A few meetings preceding the program were devoted to teaching the children the exercises.
  A precondition for participating in the study was the ability to perform the exercises perfectly
- Once a month, the children were diagnosed individually in order to monitor the status of the scoliosis and to introduce changes in the exercise program as needed
- One of the aims of the therapeutic exercises was to create high body awareness among the patients. To this end, the children were urged to modify incorrect movement patterns and make proper and efficient use of their body in daily activities.

These changes in the research design affected the results (Figs 4.16, 4.17). Comprehensive examinations after five months of treatment found that the activity had produced significant improvement in the children's status. These improvements could be seen both in scoliotic values (the COBB angles) and in a redressing of various functional asymmetries (ranges of motion) (Solberg, 1996a).

The positive effects of adapted exercise for the treatment of scoliosis were also described by Schroth (1992), who indicated that quality individual work might also bring about significant improvement.

The results of these studies indicate that therapeutic exercise may actually produce improvement in the scoliosis and engender significant change both in body posture and in general functioning of the spinal column.

The main objective of these studies was to show the possible effect of a personalized, guided therapeutic program of remedial exercise on the scoliotic spinal column. The intention was not to "prove" specific scientific facts but rather to emphasize the positive potential inherent in such a program for restoring muscular balance along the torso and reducing the degree of the disorder, if exercise intensity and quality are appropriate.

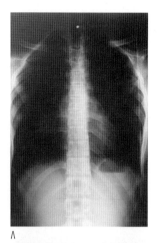

A

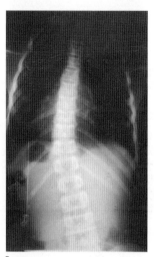

B

Figure 4.17 Comparison of X-rays (A) after treatment and (B) before treatment.

Principles for movement treatment of scoliosis

The approach presented above advocates physical exercise as part of the treatment program for scoliosis. In light of the above, such treatment must focus on many physical components, and should be conducted by trained individuals only and under close medical supervision.

To preclude possible injury resulting from improper exercise, it should be noted that realistic treatment objectives should be defined and typical contraindications in the treatment of scoliosis considered. The following are important considerations therapists should keep in mind when working with this complex disorder:

- Defining realistic therapy goals:
  In general, suitable physical activity can be of great benefit when treating scoliosis. At the same time, exercise alone cannot "correct" the disorder and "straighten" the spinal column in many instances of structural scoliosis. Therefore, the proper and responsible definition of treatment aims should entail a number of stages:
  Stage 1: Slowing the rate of scoliosis progression (during the growth period)
  Stage 2: Stopping scoliosis from progressing
  Stage 3: Improving spinal column position by reducing the scoliotic angle of deviation (if the severity of the disorder allows this)
- Consideration of rapid physical changes during the period of growth spurt:
  The literature shows that scoliosis has a tendency to develop during the body's growth spurt (Taylor, 1983; Loncar et al., 1991). This factor has important implications for monitoring the development of the disorder, and therapists must be aware of rapid physical changes during the treatment period.

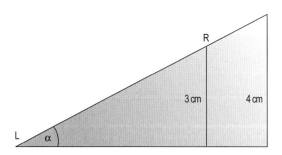

Figure 4.18 Asymmetry at scapular height.

In this context, one of the factors limiting our ability to determine the true effect of therapeutic exercise on scoliosis is the lack of reliable, accurate tests that will preclude the drawing of erroneous conclusions (Fig. 4.18).

As can be seen in Figure 4.18, taller children manifest greater asymmetry in the height of the right scapula (R) and the left scapula (L), mainly as a result of body structure. Children with broader shoulders evidence greater asymmetry than do children of the same height with narrower shoulders. This is only an optical illusion.

For this reason, objective tests are recommended (see Figs 4.10, 4.19) that will allow therapists to define asymmetry at shoulder height as the "angle of deviation" independent of individual physical dimensions. In Figure 4.18, for example, angle α is identical despite significant differences in the absolute height of the scapulae.

During their growth spurt, children may grow in height and/or breadth with no change in the angle of asymmetry. The result may be the mistaken impression that the imbalance has worsened while in fact there may even have been an improvement (Fig. 4.19).

Therefore, angle α describes asymmetry at the scapula level quite accurately, and serves as an independent measure not contingent upon a given child's physical development. One of the aims of treatment in this case is to decrease angle α to zero (balance at shoulder level), and the changes caused by body growth do not affect the results.

- Working on body awareness, changing faulty movement patterns and instilling correct movement habits. This is one of the most important aspects of treating postural disorders in general, and especially in cases of scoliosis
- Caution not to work excessively on spinal flexibility. Over-flexibility in cases of scoliosis may further damage the posture of the spine.

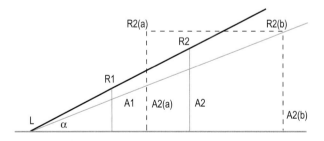

Figure 4.19 Angle of asymmetry (α) in the shoulder girdle. L–R1, first measurement (at diagnosis); L–R2, after 1 year, A2>A1, but angle is unchanged; L–R2(a), after 1 year, A2(a)>A1, but angle has increased; L–R2(b), after 1 year, A2(b)>A1, but angle has decreased.

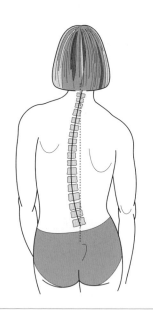

Figure 4.20 Left C-type scoliosis, for which the exercises in this chapter have been adapted.

Sample exercises

- All movement treatment of scoliosis should be conducted only by trained, qualified individuals and under the supervision of an orthopedist. Movement therapy utilizes several types of exercises. Because each case of scoliosis requires individual planning and special adaptation of exercises, one set will not necessarily be appropriate for another, even similar, case. The types, starting points, and manner of performing these exercises are adapted specifically to each person.

Types of exercises for scoliosis

1. Symmetrical exercises aimed to strengthen back and abdominal muscles and for functional improvement in ranges of joint motion.
2. Breathing exercises to increase lung volume and thorax mobility and flexibility.
3. Asymmetrical exercises for lengthening muscles on the concave (shortened) side, and for contracting muscles on the convex (lengthened) side. Asymmetrical exercises are also designed to encourage specific movement of spinal column vertebrae in desired directions (mainly for moderating or balancing rotation in cases of structural scoliosis).
4. Static exercises which also make use of body weight (various "hanging" and traction exercises) for releasing tension along the spine (see Ch. 8).

Asymmetrical exercise for scoliosis The exercises presented here are for illustration purposes only. They are adapted for a left C-type functional scoliosis (with no rotation), so that the curvature tends to the right and the right shoulder is lower than the left (Fig. 4.20).

It must be emphasized again that exercise of this sort, as treatment for scoliosis, should be performed only under professional guidance and with medical supervision, as any mistake in the direction of the exercises may worsen the situation.

Exercises for left C-type (functional) scoliosis

1. Lying face down – Right arm in straight line continuation of body, left arm beside the body.

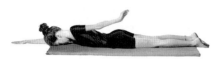 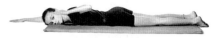

   a. Right arm is stretched forward, left shoulder is lifted from the floor and left scapula is adducted towards spinal column.

   b. Left scapula is brought towards spinal column with elbow flexed.

2. "Sleeping position" on stomach – Right arm is in straight line continuation of body, left arm flexed in front of face, right cheek on the floor, and left knee flexed to abdomen. Left scapula is adducted to spinal column and arm is lifted from the floor.

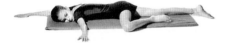 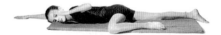

3. Face down – Right arm is straight forward, left hand under forehead.

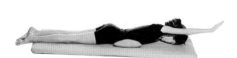 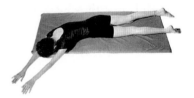

   a. Right hand and left leg are stretched in opposite directions.

   b. Right hand is moved in an "arc" to the left side, and right side of torso is stretched (position is held for a number of breaths)

4. Standing on hands and knees – Pelvis is brought to ankles. This symmetrical static stretch position is held for a number of breaths.

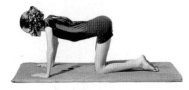 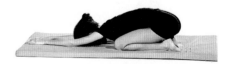

Figure 4.21 Exercises for left C-type (functional) scoliosis.

5. Standing on hands and knees – While exhaling, back is arched upwards. Pelvis is lowered to heels and forehead to the floor, while both arms are stretched forward.

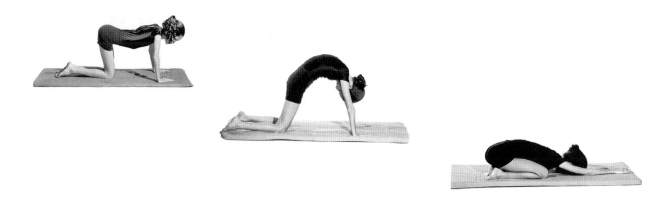

6. Lying on back – Right arm is stretched back in continuation of body line.

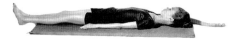

a. A deep breath is taken (inhalation).
b. While breath is held, abdominal and lower pelvic muscles are contracted while lower back is pressed towards the floor and posterior pelvic tilt is performed.
c. Breath is released, and muscular tension is released throughout body.

7. Sitting in a crossed leg position – With left hand on floor behind back and right arm extended upward, torso is tilted to left and returned to center.

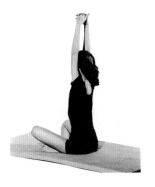 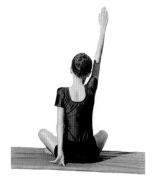 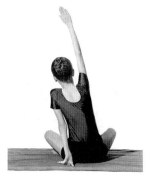

Figure 4.21 (*continued*).

8. Sitting with legs to the side, both knees facing right, both arms are abducted to the sides to shoulder height and then returned to starting position.

9. Standing, with knees slightly flexed, posterior pelvic tilt is performed and right arm is extended straight up overhead.

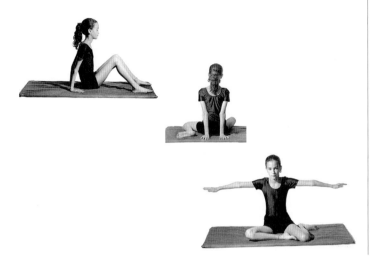
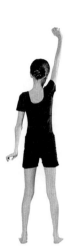
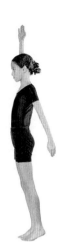

10. A number of symmetrical positions may be taken to improve body organization and spinal column on the medial line, as in the following illustrations:

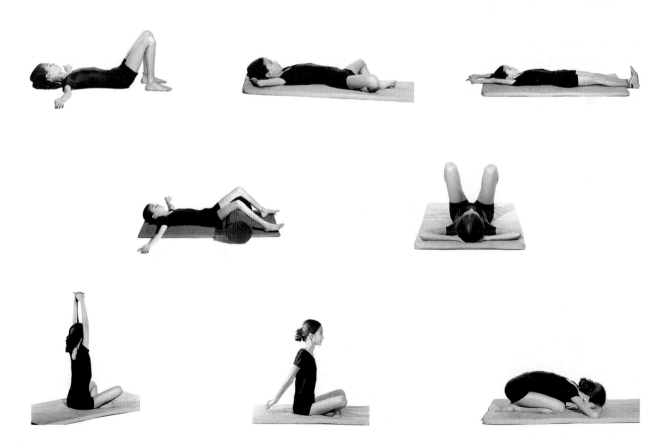

Figure 4.21 (*continued*).

CHAPTER 5

Postural disorders in the lower extremities and the identification of gait disorders

The feet provide the base for body posture as they support the entire body, and facilitate and maintain balance during activities such as standing, walking, or running.

Arches – one longitudinal and the other transverse – constitute an essential structural configuration of the foot (see Ch. 2). The alignment of bones, ligaments and muscles that maintains this structure both endows the foot with a flexibility that improves shock absorption and increases strength (Gould & Davies, 1985).

As in a chain reaction, defects in foot position may generate postural disorders higher in the body and also hamper optimal functioning of the entire body.

This chapter will survey common postural disorders of the lower extremities, focusing on problems in the feet, ankles, knees, and hips. This will be followed by a discussion of the kinesiology of walking (gait analysis) and initial diagnosis of normal walking pattern disorders.

Disorders in the lower extremities

Pes planus (flat foot)

The moment you discover which foot is your right foot, you don't have many hesitations about which of them is the left foot. And then the only problem left is which of them to start walking with ...
(A. A. Milne)

This disorder refers to a condition in which the longitudinal arch of the foot is lower than normal (Fig. 5.1). When the arch is very low, the foot lies completely flat on the standing surface, inspiring the name "flat foot".

Many cases of pes planus are also marked by foot pronation, a state in which the talus protrudes medially and increases the contact area of the foot with the ground (Fig. 5.1).

Flat foot impairs the body's shock absorption mechanism and creates motor difficulties in functions or activities requiring balance and stability. Hyperpronation may also have functional chain reaction effects throughout the lower extremities, the pelvis and the back. This is related to the subtalar joint which, during walking, transmits rotational moments to the lower extremity through its connection to the ankle joint (Norkin & Levangie, 1993).

In the gait cycle, the subtalar joint moves minimally when the foot is on the ground. Heel strike on the ground creates a neutral state. Mid-stance is marked by joint pronation (through the talus), and at the end of the movement, in push-off, the foot goes into slight supination as it pushes against the ground.

Thus, in the gait cycle the tibia responds to pronation of the subtalar joint with internal rotation and to supination with external rotation. Obviously, then, a functionally imbalanced subtalar joint will indirectly affect all the structures and joints above it, and in general, disrupt the normal walking cycle (in those stages of the walking cycle in which the foot is on the ground) (Norkin & Levangie, 1993). Details of all the stages of the walking cycle are described later in this chapter.

Flat foot is a disorder that may result from several factors:

- Structural misconfiguration of the foot bones
- Impaired functioning of the supportive ligaments of the foot joints (because of hyperflexibility)
- Weakness of intrinsic muscles that help to maintain the foot arches
- Genetic factors
- Hypermobility of the subtalar joint.

This type of disorder may also result from improper use of the foot and incorrect gait patterns.

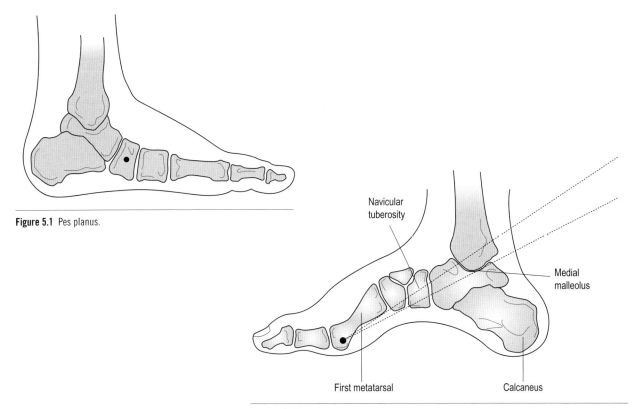

Figure 5.1 Pes planus.

Figure 5.2 Pes cavus.

Therapeutic exercise to strengthen the foot arches

Since flat foot involves structural problems, foot position may be irreparable. However, it is recommended that treatment include movement exercises. Exercises for flat foot should concentrate on:

- Strengthening the intrinsic muscles that help to maintain the foot arches
- Strengthening the muscles that perform plantar flexion.

Examples of exercises for strengthening the foot arches are described in Chapter 8.

Pes cavus (increased arches)

This disorder is characterized by increased foot arch height and usually by inversion of the subtalar joint as well. High arch is a less common disorder than flat foot. Because of the heightened arch, foot contact with the ground is smaller than normal, thus creating an unbalanced weight distribution. As a result, existing support points are subjected to greater pressures from loads bearing down on them (Fig. 5.2). Over-inversion may also impair the foot's ability to adjust to different surfaces while walking (Norkin & Levangie, 1993).

The main treatment for this disorder is orthopedic, with special shoe inserts adapted to the foot to provide support by filling in the extra space created by the condition. At the same time, movement can be integrated in the form of exercises to improve foot joint mobility and flexibility.

*For methods of measuring and evaluating foot arches see Chapter 2, Figures 2.7, 2.8

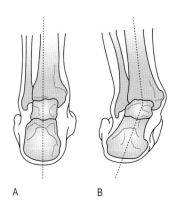

Figure 5.3 Posterior view of left foot. (A) Normal. (B) Pes valgus (pronated foot).

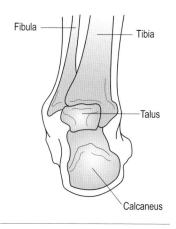

Figure 5.4 Posterior view of left foot. Pes varus (supinated foot).

Pes valgus (pronated foot)

Because the structural formation of the ankle joint facilitates movement mainly on the sagittal plane (plantar and dorsi-flexion) (see Ch. 2), pes valgus with its concomitant eversion occurs in essence in the foot, in the joint between the talus bone and the calcaneus bones (subtalar joint) (Kahle et al., 1986).

This disorder is characterized by a "sinking" of the medial border of the foot to a low flat position, which exposes its lateral border to excess loads (Fig. 5.3).

As most cases of pronated foot are related to flat foot, the kinesiological aspects and functional disorders created by pes valgus are described in the section on flat foot.

Pes varus (supinated foot)

In this condition, which is the reverse of pes valgus or pronated foot, the foot is in a state of inversion and most of the load is exerted on the medial border of the foot (Fig. 5.4).

Movement treatment for pronated/supinated feet

Both of these foot position disorders can be improved somewhat by appropriate treatment that emphasizes the following:

- Learning and exercising balanced body alignment on all of the foot support points (see Ch. 9)
- Basing and rooting exercises, combined with resistance techniques applied by the therapist (as also described in Ch. 9)
- Exercises for strengthening the foot arches (see Ch. 8).

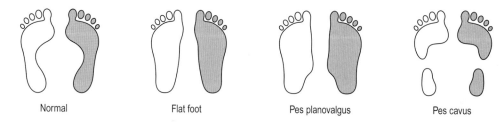

Figure 5.5 Disorders of the foot.

Genu valgum (knock knees)

This disorder of the knee position is characterized by the closeness to one another of the two medial femoral condyles (Fig. 5.6). The result is an imbalanced distribution of weight on the knee joint and extra loads and wear on the lateral aspect of the joint. The cause of genu valgum is usually structural in nature, but it may also be part of a chain reaction to foot eversion (pes valgus).

Genu varum (bowlegs)

This disorder is characterized by a greater than usual distance between the knees in an erect position. Here, weight distribution on the tibia surfaces is imbalanced, with the medial aspect of the knee bearing the main load (Kahle et al., 1986) (Fig. 5.7). In addition to structural causes, genu varum is often the result of inverted foot position (pes varus).

The effectiveness of movement therapy in many cases of genu varum or genu valgum is limited because of the structural nature of the problem. However, if the problem originates in incorrect foot position, treatment can focus on improving foot placement, as described in the sections on pronated/supinated foot.

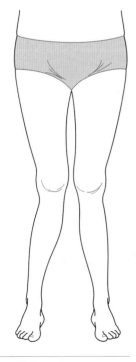

Figure 5.6 Genu valgum.

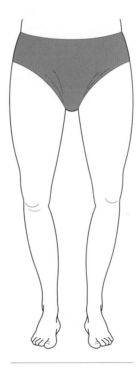

Figure 5.7 Genu varum.

Structural effects of the femur on knee joint position

Another factor affecting knee joint position is the anatomical structure of the femur, especially the angle created between the femur shaft and neck (the neck shaft angle) (Fig. 5.8). In infants, this angle measures about 150° and over the years, it decreases to about 120° as a result of life cycle changes (Gould & Davies, 1985; Kahle et al., 1986).

The neck shaft angle impacts on the relationship between the femur shaft and the line of gravity that passes through the lower extremities. In normal conditions, the line of gravity passes directly from the center of the femur head, through the center of the knee, to the center of the heel. Changes in neck shaft angle may cause changes in leg position: a smaller than normal angle will create genu valgum (knock knees) and a larger than normal angle will produce genu varum (bowlegs) (Fig. 5.9). This explains why infants are characterized by bowlegs in their early stages of development.

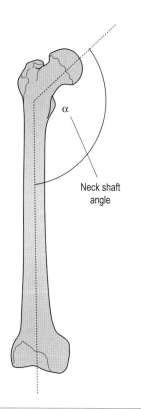

Figure 5.8 Neck shaft angle of the femur bone.

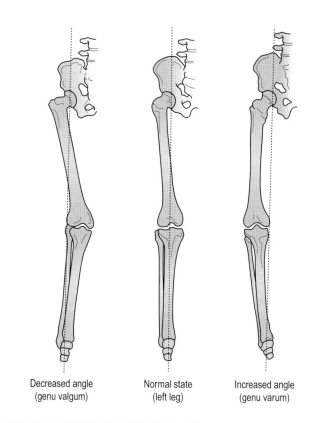

Decreased angle   Normal state   Increased angle
(genu valgum)   (left leg)   (genu varum)

Figure 5.9 Influence of neck shaft angle of the femur on lower extremity position.

Tibial torsion

This rotational condition in the tibia is usually diagnosed by means of observation from the front (Fig. 5.10). When both feet point straight ahead, one or both knees face inward or outward. Alternatively, when both knees point straight ahead, the feet turn out or in (toes out – toes in). In other words, this disorder is characterized by rotation of the tibia in relation to the femur.

The cause of tibial torsion is usually related to bone structure, thus limiting the effectiveness of movement treatment. Because of the torsion created in the knee joint, inappropriate exercise may be harmful. In all such cases, treatment should be carried out under close medical supervision.

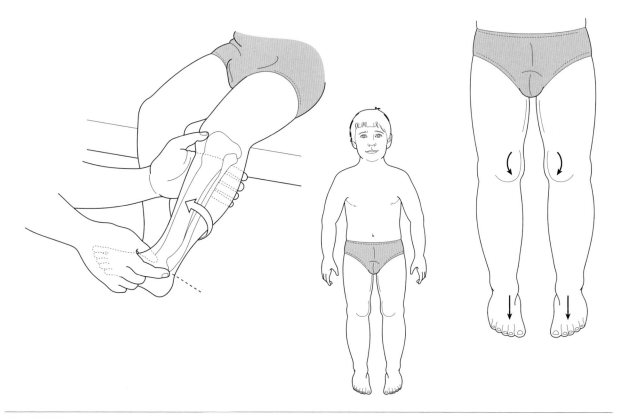

Figure 5.10 Tibial torsion.

Changes in femoral torsion angle

Another factor tracing back to the anatomical structure of the femur may also affect the angle between feet. This is the torsion angle. Femoral torsion angle refers to the relationship between the longitudinal line of the femur neck and the line connecting the two femoral condyles (Fig. 5.11).

Under normal conditions, torsion angle in adults is 12°, and it is responsible in part for transforming hip flexion in such a way that rotational movements of the femur head fit into the acetabulum (Kahle et al., 1986). Changes in the torsion angle may produce postural problems in the lower extremities. An angle >12° (anteversion) will be indicated by a toe-in position of the feet, while a smaller than normal angle (retroversion – <12°) will create a toe-out position (Norkin & Levangie, 1993).

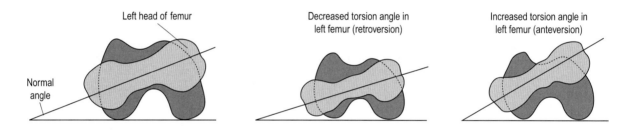

Figure 5.11 Torsion angle (for left femur, view from above).

Genu recurvatum (hyperextension of the knee)

Hyperextension of the knee is diagnosable through observation from the side. In a normal standing position the knee joint is characterized by extension. Regular functioning of the ligaments and muscles enveloping the knee provides good support and stability, and prevents the joint from hyperextension, thus limiting its movement backwards.

When this support is compromised by weakness of the soft tissues or by structural problems, the result is hyperextension – movement beyond the normal extension range. In this condition, the joint shifts from its normal position and overloads the anterior aspect of the knee (Fig. 5.12).

In turn, as part of a chain reaction, the change in knee position disrupts both the ankle joint position (below the knee) and the pelvic position (above it), undermining optimal balance for the entire body.

Movement treatment of knee hyperextension focuses on two elements:

1. Exercises to strengthen the muscles enveloping and stabilizing the knee joint.
2. Work on physical awareness and altering movement patterns of the lower extremities.

Focusing only on muscle-strengthening treatment will often yield less-than-satisfactory results because most disorders of this type are structurally generated. Therefore, the most important emphasis in treatment should be on learning and practicing new movement patterns that prevent, as much as can be obtained, knee hyperextension. The resistance techniques described in Chapter 9 are especially effective in this regard.

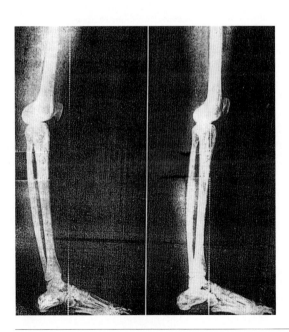

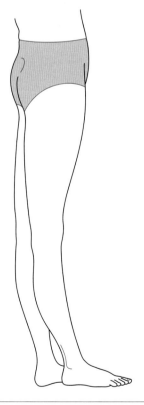

Figure 5.12 Genu recurvatum (hyperextension).

Identification of functional gait disorders

Biomechanical aspects and gait principles

A variety of postural disorders are reflected in deviant walking patterns. Diagnosing walking patterns is an important component of the general diagnosis of posture, which in this context refers to general body functioning in dynamic situations.

This section will focus on the basic gait (movement) characteristics in order to help diagnose disorders in this mode of locomotion. Because this book is intended mainly for therapists, emphasis has been placed on the aspects most important to their clinical work (without providing an extended analysis of each gait component).

Gait analysis

Walking is defined as a linear (straight) progression, which is attained through coordinated movements of the body joints and transfer of the center of gravity from place to place. The gait analysis presented here treats one gait cycle as representative of the entire gait action.

A gait cycle is defined as an action that commences the moment one foot touches the ground and ends when that same foot touches the ground again. The initial point of foot contact with the ground is

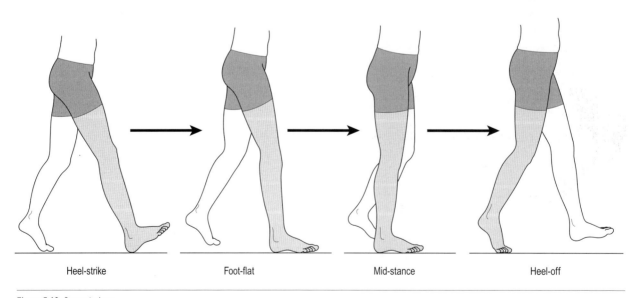

| Heel-strike | Foot-flat | Mid-stance | Heel-off |

Figure 5.13 Support phase.

usually considered the beginning of a walking cycle. Although this cycle takes only about 1 second, it encompasses many body actions. Thus walking analysis necessitates the processing of tremendous amounts of information in a short time, for which high level skill and extensive experience are required. It is also recommended that diagnosticians analyze video recordings of the walking process under controlled conditions (and if necessary, review the recordings in regular and slow motion).

The walking cycle is composed of two main stages (Figs 5.13, 5.14):

1. *The support phase*, in which one foot is in contact with the ground.
2. *The swing phase*, in which the same foot is propelled forward after it pushes off, in preparation for a new cycle.

The support phase comprises about 60% of the overall duration of each cycle, with the swing phase accounting for the remaining 40%. It is also clear that during part of each cycle both feet are in contact with the ground simultaneously, creating double support. The faster the walking pace, the shorter will be the double-support time span, down to zero time, i.e. when the body shifts from walking to running.

Stride length is defined as the distance between the initial contact of one foot (e.g., the right heel) and the initial contact of the second foot (the left foot in this example). A cycle is defined as two consecutive steps that include the support phase and the swing phase.

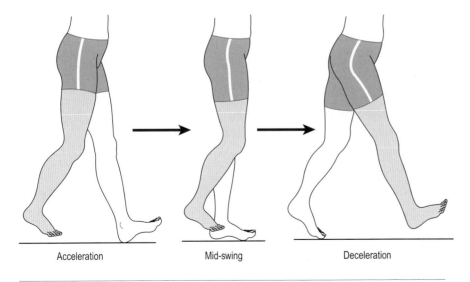

Acceleration   Mid-swing   Deceleration

Figure 5.14 Swing phase.

The support phase is made up of a number of stages *(Fig. 5.13)*

1. Heel-strike – commencement of the walking cycle, when the heel contacts the ground.
2. Foot-flat – when the whole foot is in full contact with the ground.
3. Mid-stance – the stage in which the body's center of gravity passes over the base of the stepping area.
4. Heel-off – lifting the heel from the ground while rising on the toes.
5. Toes-off – disconnecting the toes from the ground.

Swing phase *(Fig. 5.14)*

This phase of the walking cycle includes a forward shifting of the foot that has just completed its contact with the ground, in a forward rotational movement.

This phase can be divided into three stages:

1. Acceleration: from the moment the foot disconnects from the ground halfway through the swing phase arc.
2. Mid-swing: half route of the foot-shifting towards the ground.
3. Deceleration: from half of the route to heel touching point with the ground.

Important points to note in diagnosing walking disorders

General leg functioning

Leg thrust against the ground creates the force that moves the body forward, assisted by flexible movements of the ankle, knee, and hip joints. How much time both feet are in contact with the ground simultaneously depends on stride frequency. It is advisable to monitor whether strides maintain consistency in terms of rhythm and length.

Foot and ankle position during walking

- Examining coronal/frontal plane disorders in the feet and ankles (during walking)
  - Pronated foot (pes valgus)
  - Supinated foot (pes varus)
- Explanations of pronated/supinated foot appear in the sections discussing foot disorders at the beginning of this chapter
- Movement quality in the sagittal plane (dorsi-flexion – plantar flexion).

Ankle flexion and extension are connected to knee and hip movements. Movement in the ankle joint provides good shock absorption and stability in the stepping stage and moves the body forward in the final stage of push off from the ground.

Functional impairment to these ranges of motion on the sagittal plane – whether because of muscle shortness or muscular weakness – will appear as disorders in heel-to-toe foot rolling, which will impair walking function as a whole. Two common disorders may appear in this part of the cycle:

Toe walking Functional shortening of the plantar flexor muscles performing plantar flexion may cause a raised-heel gait pattern (toe walking) and difficulty in the heel-strike stage (this walking pattern is characteristic of cerebral palsy in cases of shortened Achilles tendon).

Toe walking may be the result of factors other than shortened muscles, such as wrong movement patterns, motor control difficulties, or postural problems due to emotional issues (mainly among young children).

Drop foot Functional weakness of the dorsi-flexion muscles may cause the foot to drop so that the toes touch the ground before the heel (Fig. 5.15).

During the heel-strike stage, dorsi-flexion in the foot stretches the Achilles tendon, enhancing knee stability during the straightening performed while stepping on the heel. Therefore, in cases of drop foot, the foot both hits the ground and weakens the knee joint. To examine foot position, it is recommended to test walking bare-footed as well.

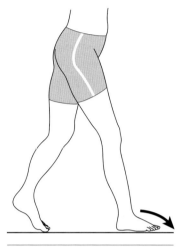

Figure 5.15 Drop foot in walking.

Knee joint position during walking

- Genu valgum (knock knees)
- Genu varum (bowlegs).

Width of support base during walking

Body stability during walking is affected by the dimensions of the support base and the distance between the feet.

In standing, the person's two feet form the body's support base, with the line of gravity passing between them (in the center of the base of support). Thus feet that are slightly open provide better stability.

However, while walking the support base shifts from leg to leg, and to maintain stability, the body's center of gravity must also shift and cross over the base of support – above the supporting leg.

If a person's legs move straight forward from a static standing position (walking with a large leg span), body weight must shift considerably from side to side with each step. It is possible to create the effect of this type of walking by standing with feet spread slightly, trying to lift one leg at a time and then returning it to the same place. This effort produces a lateral movement of the entire body in order to maintain balance. Thus, walking with a broad base of support creates a "duck walk" movement pattern – with the body waddling from side to side. This is the movement pattern characteristic of babies' first stages of walking. This extra distance between their legs enhances body stability and maintains balance.

One way of preventing duck walk swaying is by placing each foot closer to the center of gravity with each step (walking on a straight line and placing each foot directly in front of the other). However, the disadvantage of this type of walking is that it decreases the body's support base in the double support phase (when both feet are in contact with the ground), thus reducing body stability. Moreover, energy is wasted in shifting the foot laterally to bypass the second leg with each step.

The most effective foot position in walking is one that minimizes side-to-side swaying, while allowing the leg to move directly forward. In this position, the medial (inner) borders of the feet almost touch a straight line during walking. The support base area will be somewhat wider than in walking on a straight line, but the feet can move directly forward, and side-to-side movement of the body's center of gravity will be reduced to a minimum (Figs 5.16, 5.17).

To summarize, walking on an excessively broad support base (too great a span between feet) may indicate difficulties in dynamic balance. In such cases, it is recommended to specifically examine balance ability (see Ch. 7).

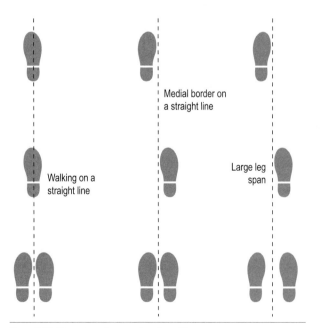

Walking on a straight line

Medial border on a straight line

Large leg span

Figure 5.16 Dimensions of support base in walking.

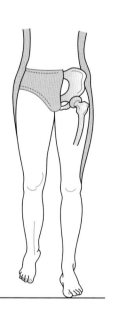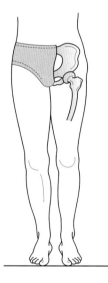

Figure 5.17 Minimal movement of the center of gravity from side to side.

In contrast, a narrow walking base allows the body to lean on the weight-carrying leg, thus reducing movement of the center of gravity in the walking cycle, which allows smooth, effective and efficient movements with less energy (Fig. 5.18).

Angle between feet

Another important aspect to monitor is toe direction. The feet roll parallel in normal walking, like wheels on a rail. They roll from the center of the heel on the central axis of the foot to the five toes. Where a prominent angle between the feet is visible, normal walking function may be impaired in two possible ways:

1. Toe-out position (a "Charlie Chaplin" walk).
2. Toe-in position – legs may touch during walking, with a concomitant tendency to fall.

Walking with toes pointed straight ahead directs the locomotion thrust in the exact walking direction desired. If feet toe-out or in (because of postural problems), the thrust is oblique (Fig. 5.19) and may cause other problems:

- Excessive energy expenditure in walking
- Unbalanced "zig-zag" walking
- Pressure points on various parts of the foot which subject them to accelerated wear.

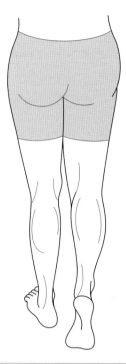

Figure 5.18 A small distance (a few cm) between feet that still allows a reasonable base of support.

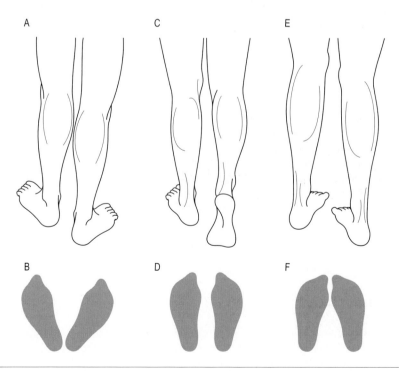

Figure 5.19 Angle variations between the feet in walking. (A,B) toe-out; (C,D) toe straight forward; (E,F) toe-in.

Each of the above conditions can be traced back to any of a number of possible causes, such as changes in the femoral torsion angle (Fig. 5.11) or functional asymmetry in hip or knee joint position. Therefore, it is advisable to examine these joints in terms of anatomical position, ranges of motion and balance between the antagonistic muscle groups surrounding them. It is also recommended to examine the joints for possible functional imbalance because of structural problems.

Arm movements

Forward and backward movements of the arms close to the body assist in body balance. Movement flow in cases of normal coordination entails movement of right arm with left leg, and vice versa. Coordinative disorders may be visible in parallel movement (arm and leg on the same side); these can disrupt movement flow and balance.

Pelvic function

As for pelvic functioning in walking, examination should concentrate on the movements of the pelvis in the following:

Pelvic rotation In the walking cycle, rotational movement is created on the transverse (horizontal) plane of the pelvis when the foot is in the air in the swing phase accompanying pelvic rotation. The momentum that is produced carries the pelvis forward, and this in turn affects the amplitude of the rise and fall of the center of gravity along the movement path.

Pelvic tilt The pelvis on the side of the raised leg (in the swing phase) tends to fall (Fig. 5.20). The muscle action on the side of the supporting leg (mainly the action of the gluteus medius muscle), together with contraction of the quadratus lumborum on the opposite side, prevents this fall and facilitates pelvic balance.

Common characteristics of walking disorders

Table 5.1 Salient and common gait disorders and their possible sources

OBSERVED CHARACTERISTICS	POSSIBLE CAUSES (TO BE CHECKED)
1 Improper movement flow. Unilateral movement of the legs and arms (no movement of opposing arm/leg). Heavy steps, rigid movement patterns.	Motor clumsiness Coordinative disorders
2 Walking with a broad support base, large span between legs. Body rocks from side to side in movement.	Difficulties maintaining balance Lack of hip joint stability
3 Knee or foot contact (or rubbing) while walking. Tendency to fall often.	Disorders in ankle, knee or hip joint position Contractures of adductor muscles and weakness of hip abduction muscles
4 "Sloppy" walking. Rubbing or 'dragging' feet on ground.	Low body awareness Movement habits Relaxed posture Overall weakness
5 Excessive movement of pelvis towards the weight-bearing leg.	Functional weakness of gluteus medius. Trendelenburg syndrome (see Fig. 5.20)
6 Asymmetry in pelvic movement and imbalance in pelvic height. One side appears lower in each stage of walking.	Scoliosis Unequal leg length Functional imbalance of antagonist muscles around hip joint (see Ch. 2, Fig. 2.17)
7 Drop foot (toes touch ground before heel) (see Fig. 5.15)	Functional weakness of muscles performing dorsiflexion
8 High heel walking. Difficulty placing heel on ground during heel strike phase.	Functional shortening/contraction of muscles performing plantar flexion (shortening of Achilles tendon)
9 Toe-in	Tibial torsion Torsion angle of hip bone is >12° Imbalance of hip joints Muscular imbalance – shortening of internal hip rotators or weakness of external hip rotators
10 Toe-out	Tibial torsion Decreased torsion angle of hip bone (<12°) Imbalance of hip joints Muscular imbalance – shortening of external hip rotators

Identifying functional gait disorders

The best way to identify and diagnose walking disorders is by recording the patient's gait on a video tape and later to observe his walking, as recorded, at the therapist's leisure (preferably in slow motion). In most cases, initial identification of problems is necessary in "real time", while watching the child walk (as part of the overall diagnostic process). Table 5.1 details a few of the salient and common disorders as well as their possible sources. It does not mention severe disorders caused by physical problems entailing neural damage. It should also be kept in mind that each symptom or characteristic presented in this section can have many causes, not all of which are mentioned. Therefore, therapists must examine each case individually and not make snap diagnoses.

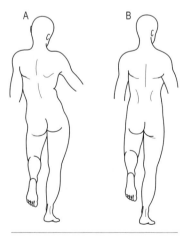

Figure 5.20 (A) Functional weakness of gluteus medius muscle (Trendelenburg syndrome). (B) Normal condition.

CHAPTER 6

Postural disorders and musculoskeletal dysfunction in the upper extremities

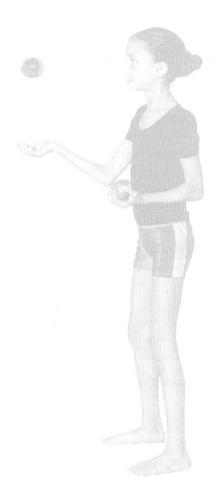

The interaction of static components and dynamic muscle tendons allows the shoulder girdle to move multidirectionally on all planes. Normal movement is a result of the balanced and synchronized action of all joints and movement centers connected to the shoulder, in coordination with the spinal joints in the cervical and thoracic vertebrae (Kamkar et al., 1993) (see Ch. 2).

Many shoulder girdle movements create functional chain reactions in adjacent joints, specially the spine. Conversely, spinal position and the functioning of all the joints along the spine affect shoulder position.

Preceding chapters have mentioned conditions in which faulty spinal position indirectly affects shoulder girdle functioning (see Kyphosis in Ch. 2). This chapter will focus on common disorders in the shoulder girdle area and their indirect effect on spinal functioning.

The contents of this chapter are based on the anatomical and kinesiological background material about the shoulder girdle presented in Chapter 2. However, due to the functional complexity of this area, additional kinesiological information not mentioned before has been introduced into this chapter.

Stabilizing elements of the shoulder girdle

In most daily activities, the joints of the upper extremity usually do not have to bear great weight, and the evolutionary result has been alterations that in effect "sacrifice" joint stability in order to gain greater movement ranges. The consequence of this anatomical change in structure of the shoulder joint is a characteristic instability, as the articulated surface in the glenoid cavity in the scapula is very flat and not adapted to the rounded structure of the humeral head.

The osseous structure of the joint is defined as a multiaxial ball and socket in which the humeral head is four times as large as the glenoid cavity, so that only part of the humeral head is in contact with the glenoid cavity at any given joint position. Nevertheless, the shoulder joint succeeds in maintaining stability by means of passive and active systems working synergetically (Fig. 6.1). The passive system includes several structures that work statically, and they, in essence, serve as the primary stabilizers of the shoulder. The active system includes the rotator cuff muscles, which interlock with the capsule and impart dynamic stability to the joint (Hess, 2000).

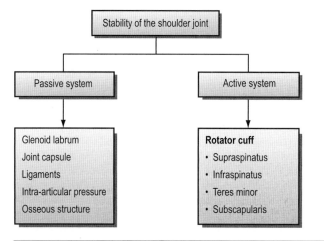

Figure 6.1 Passive and active systems that contribute to stabilizing the shoulder joint.

The elements stabilizing the shoulder joint

The glenoid labrum *(Fig. 6.2)*

This cartilaginous casing is located around the glenoid cavity, and contributes to greater shoulder stability by slightly deepening the joint.

Capsuloligamentous mechanism *(Fig. 6.3)*

The capsule, together with a number of ligaments, contributes to joint stability. It begins from the borders of the glenoid cavity in the scapula and reaches the anatomical neck of the humerus. When the arm is hanging in its natural anatomical position, the upper half of the humeral head comes in contact with the capsule, and the bottom half comes in contact with the glenoid cavity.

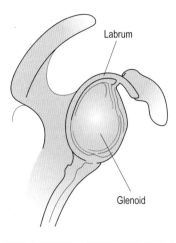

Figure 6.2 Glenoid labrum.

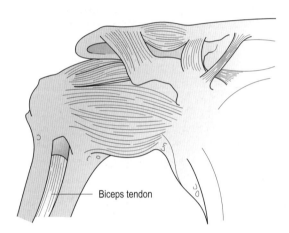

Figure 6.3 Shoulder capsule, anterior view.

The capsule plays an important role in stabilizing the shoulder, especially at the "extremes" of the ranges of motion, so that during lateral rotation of the arm the anterior part of the capsule is stretched, and during medial rotation its rear part is stretched (Kahle et al., 1986).

Supporting ligaments *(Fig. 6.4)*

The ligaments connecting the various structures attached to the shoulder are extremely important for joint stability, as they limit excessive movement in all planes. These are the main ligaments that stabilize the shoulder:

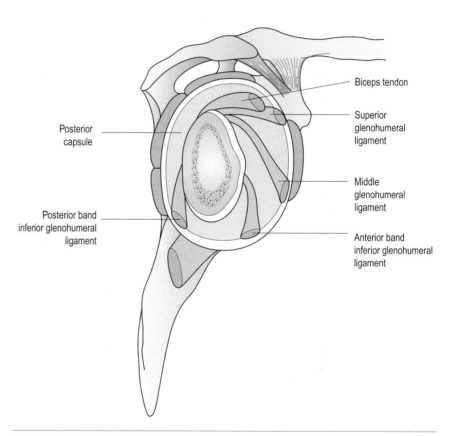

Biceps tendon

Superior glenohumeral ligament

Middle glenohumeral ligament

Anterior band inferior glenohumeral ligament

Posterior capsule

Posterior band inferior glenohumeral ligament

Figure 6.4 Ligaments supporting the shoulder joint.

- *Coracohumeral ligament* – This ligament passes from the base of the coracoid process on the scapula and connects to the greater and lesser tubercles of the humerus. The ligament supports the humeral head as it resists the downward pull of gravity
- *Superior glenohumeral ligament* – The origin of this ligament is near the biceps brachii tendon and it connects slightly above the lesser tubercle of the humerus. This ligament strengthens the anterior superior wall of the capsule in the shoulder joint and prevents downward dislocation of the humeral head when the arm is hanging or is held close to the body
- *Middle glenohumeral ligament* – The origin of this ligament is somewhat medial to the lesser tubercle of the humerus and is connected to the scapula in the center of the glenoid cavity. The ligament strengthens the anterior wall of the joint capsule and limits lateral rotation of the arm. Weakness in this ligament causes instability in the anterior aspect of the joint
- *Inferior glenohumeral ligament* – The origin of this ligament is in the area of the glenoid cavity of the scapula and is connected to the anatomical neck of the humerus. This ligament strengthens the inferior anterior wall of the capsule, and in addition prevents dislocation of the humeral head from the joint socket; its anterior and posterior parts also limit internal and external rotation (respectively).

Intra-articular pressure (vacuum effect)

The rotator cuff muscles that encase the joint from all sides create a compression or vacuum effect that presses the humeral head into the glenoid cavity. Under normal conditions, this compression remains constant within the joint and contributes to its stability (Hess, 2000).

Osseous structure

The meeting of the scapula with the ribs facilitates a sliding movement along the wall of the thoracic cage, with the clavicle in front acting as a "supporting beam". This support helps to stabilize the scapula when opposing muscular forces are working on it, performing medial rotation and scapular adduction. In this way, the clavicle helps to maintain shoulder stability by means of its points of connection to the scapula and the sternum.

Stabilizing muscles

Most of the muscles affecting movement and stability of the shoulder girdle are presented in full detail in the tables of muscles in Chapter 2, with reference to their points of origin and insertion. Therefore, this chapter emphasizes only those muscle actions related specifically to the shoulder joint.

Anatomically speaking, it is possible to classify the muscles that stabilize the shoulder joint into three groups.

The superficial group

Table 6.1

MUSCLE	MUSCLE ACTION IN RELATION TO THE SHOULDER JOINT	
Deltoid	Arm abduction beyond 30° Clavicular head and posterior scapular head help in arm adduction Anterior muscle fibers also perform internal rotation from a position in which the arm is rotated externally Posterior muscle fibers also perform external rotation from a position in which the arm is rotated internally	
Coracobrachialis	Flexion of arm Adduction of arm	
Biceps brachii (long head)	Flexion of elbow (with supinated forearm) Long head participates in humeral abduction when the humerus is in lateral rotation The short head assists in humeral adduction and flexion The muscle contributes to joint stability by preventing the humeral head from slipping upward	Origin Biceps brachii Tendon Radius Ulna Insertion Humerus Scapula

Deep group (rotator cuff) Shoulder stability depends very much on the rotator cuff encasing it. The rotator cuff muscles are an important stabilizing factor that provides active support to the joint. (As noted, full anatomical details about origins and insertions of each muscle appear in the tables of muscles in Ch. 2.)

Table 6.2

MUSCLE	MUSCLE ACTION IN RELATION TO THE SHOULDER JOINT
Supraspinatus	Humeral abduction from 0–30° with slight external rotation Stabilizes the humeral head in the shoulder joint
Infraspinatus	Lateral rotation of the humerus and arm extension Stabilizes the humeral head in the shoulder joint and contributes especially to anterior stability of the joint in positions of abduction with lateral rotation
Teres minor	Lateral rotation of the humerus Stabilizes the humeral head in the shoulder joint and contributes especially to anterior stability of the joint in a state of abduction with lateral rotation
Subscapularis	Medial rotation of the humerus and humeral adduction Stabilizes the humeral head in the shoulder joint

The peripheral group

Table 6.3

MUSCLE	MUSCLE ACTION IN RELATION TO THE SHOULDER JOINT
Latissimus dorsi	Extension and adduction of the humerus in a state of flexion When the humerus is in a state of adduction it also creates medial rotation When the two sides work together they draw shoulders back and down
Pectoralis major	Adduction and medial rotation of the humerus Horizontal adduction of humerus ("hugging" movement)
Teres major	Extension, adduction and medial rotation of the humerus Synergist muscle with the latissimus dorsi

Tables 6.1–6.3 present the main muscles affecting the shoulder joint. Other muscles working on the entire shoulder girdle appear in detail in Chapter 2.

Survey of common disorders of the shoulder girdle

In various movements, the shoulder joint acts as a link between the upper extremity and the trunk, and in terms of the skeletal system, there are interrelationships between joint position and the functioning of the muscle casing enveloping these joints. Functional impairments to the shoulder girdle are quite common in the population at large, and for the most part they involve a number of limiting factors (Glousman, 1993). A problem in the shoulder girdle may be the result of faulty functioning of any of the components connected to it.

The most common disorders of the shoulder girdle

Wing scapulae

The shoulder girdle needs to provide a combination of broad range of movements and a stable base of support for the arm. The scapula plays a central role in this function as it connects all the structures affecting shoulder movement. Imbalance in the normal position of the scapula impairs functional efficiency in all the muscles acting on it, and especially in the rotator cuff, which cannot operate optimally in such a condition. Dynamic stability of the scapula requires coordinated and well-timed muscular action, and faulty muscle functioning may cause improper positioning of the scapula and impair the shoulder joint itself.

1. Anatomical and physiological aspects of postural characteristics of scapular position

   In normative conditions, scapular position forms an angle of 30° anterior to the frontal plane (Fig. 6.5). This position allows optimal movement of the arm in horizontal adduction and abduction, and

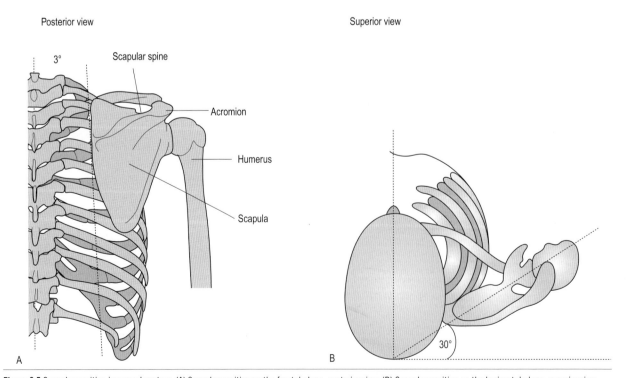

Posterior view

Superior view

3°

Scapular spine

Acromion

Humerus

Scapula

30°

A

B

Figure 6.5 Scapular position in normal posture. (A) Scapular position on the frontal plane, posterior view. (B) Scapular position on the horizontal plane, superior view.

the scapula accompanies the movement of the arm accordingly. During horizontal adduction the scapulae move apart from one another, and the angle exceeds 30° (Fig. 6.6); during horizontal abduction the angle decreases to <30°, and the scapulae draw closer to one another.

2. Common patterns of unbalanced scapular position

The broad array of movements by the shoulder girdle is made possible mainly by the combination of movement options created at the junction of the scapula and thoracic ribs (scapulothoracic articulation) with movements that are made possible in the glenohumeral joint (the shoulder joint).

The scapula should produce movement that is broad but at the same time in proper balance while also maintaining proximity to the thoracic cage. Problems of scapular movement in relation to the thorax (scapulothoracic dyskinesis) can take on a variety of patterns (Kibler et al., 2002). One of the common disorders of the scapulae is called wing scapulae, a condition in which the scapula moves away from the thoracic cage and protrudes to the rear. Scapular protrusion has a number of forms, as illustrated in Figure 6.7.

3. Factors causing impaired scapular position in wing scapulae

One of the most common causes of protrusion of the medial (vertebral) border of the scapula is weakness of the serratus anterior muscle which is responsible, among other things, for fastening the scapula to the thorax (Fig. 6.7A).

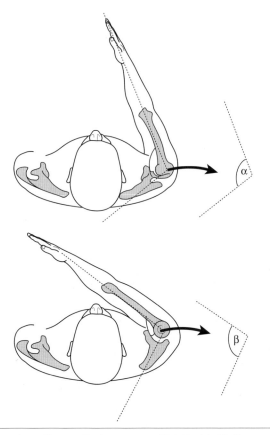

Figure 6.6 Change in scapular position according to arm movement in horizontal adduction.

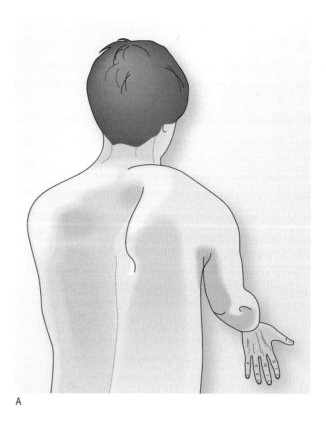

A

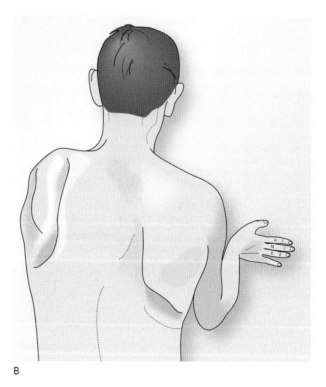

B

Figure 6.7 Wing scapulae. (A) Medial scapular winging: The medial vertebral border of the scapula moves away from the thoracic cage. The protrusion is emphasized mainly during pushing (such as against a wall) from a position of arm flexion. (B) Lateral scapular winging: The lateral vertebral border of the scapula protrudes during arm abduction.

Weakness in the trapezius muscle may also cause the scapulae to protrude in relation to the thorax, but in this case the result is lateral winging (Fig. 6.7B). The aim of movement therapy in these conditions is to improve scapular stability and to make them adhere closer to the thorax by concentrating on exercises that strengthen the trapezius and serratus anterior muscles.

Weakness in the shoulder girdle

Weakness in the shoulder girdle may affect a number of planes:

1. Faulty posture, such as slouching shoulders, rounded back and relaxed posture (see Ch. 3)
2. Difficulties in gross motor functioning that are manifested in poor movement quality and motor clumsiness. This characteristic is especially prominent in skills based on stability or on strength in the shoulder girdle, such as shooting a ball at a basket, passing a ball, hitting with a bat, etc.
3. Functional difficulties in fine motor skills and in manipulative actions employing the wrist and fingers in proximal-distal coordination patterns in motor development.

   This important pattern in motor development can be seen in the strong functional link between gross and fine motor skills. Throughout the initial stages of infant development, proximal muscles (those closer to the midline of the body) develop motor coordination and control before distal muscles (those farther from the midline of the body). Thus, stability of the proximal muscles around the shoulder girdle constitutes an essential functional basis for the use of small muscle groups in the hand.

   Weakness and instability in the shoulder girdle impede control of fine motor actions such as writing, cutting, handling a knife and fork, and regulating the precise amounts of strength applied in such actions. Many children suffering from hypotonus and weakness of the shoulder girdle exhibit difficulties in writing, often with adverse effects on their academic achievements. In these conditions, gradual strengthening of the shoulder girdle may significantly improve fine motor functioning. (This developmental aspect is described in detail in Ch. 12, which deals with postural disorders in early childhood). Examples of exercises for strengthening the shoulder girdle can be found at the end of this chapter.

   It is important to note that fine motor difficulties in children may be attributable to other factors as well, unconnected to weakness of the shoulder girdle. Such difficulties may also be caused by hypertonus of the muscles, and difficulties in precision and in strength regulation that may stem from problems in differentiating movement.

   Differentiated movement is essential for fine motor functioning and is manifested in the ability to activate each limb separately and effectively while neutralizing points of tension and muscle contraction in other body limbs (see Ch. 7). Difficulties in writing caused by this problem can be traced to a faulty functional connection between the shoulder and elbow joints, and the wrist.

In such cases, excessive strength is applied by the large muscles around the shoulder girdle and movement treatment should focus on this functional connection in order to enhance differentiated movement.

The following examples of motor activities are intended to improve differentiated movement and the functional connection among the joints of the upper extremity (shoulder–elbow–wrist) in an 8-year-old girl (Fig. 6.8)

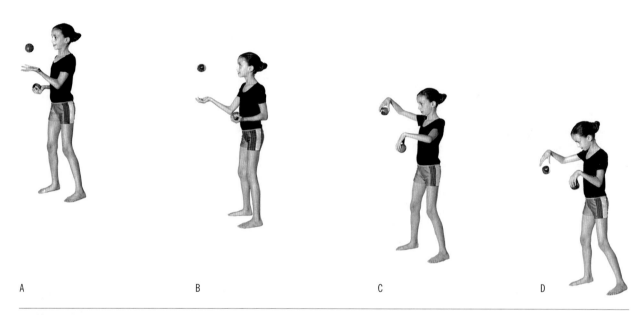

A   B   C   D

Figure 6.8A–D Variations of juggling exercises.

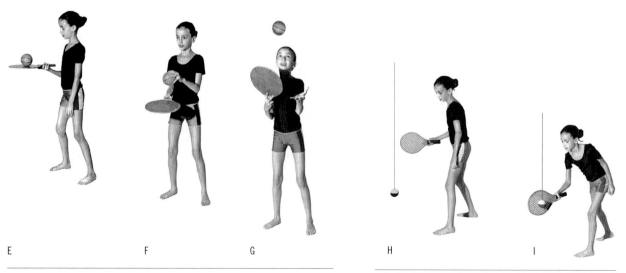

E   F   G   H   I

Figure 6.8E–G Guiding a ball on a bat.

Figure 6.8H, I Batting a string ball (with a bat).

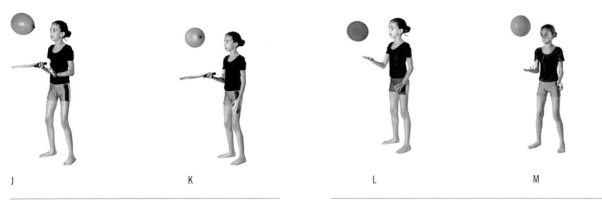

J   K   L   M

Figure 6.8J,K Batting a balloon with a bat.

Figure 6.8L,M Batting a balloon with hands.

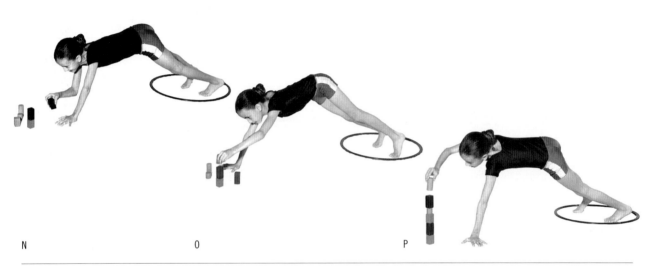

N   O   P

Figure 6.8N–P Building a tower of blocks.

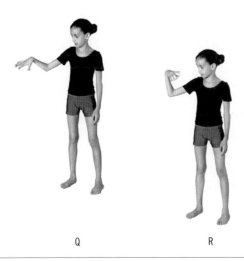

Q   R

Figure 6.8Q,R Shaking stickers off a hand (additional examples of shaking exercises are presented in Ch. 9).

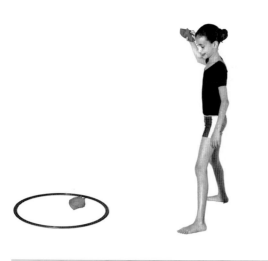

Figure 6.8S Throwing a bag at a hoop.

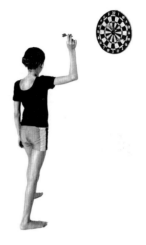

Figure 6.8T Throwing darts at a target.

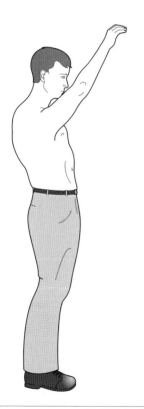

Figure 6.9 Forward movement of the pelvis as a chain reaction to weakness of the shoulder girdle when raising arms.

4. The effect of shoulder girdle weakness on the lower back

Fatigue and weakness of the axioscapular muscles (connecting the scapula and the trunk) are manifested in scapular instability mainly during arm abduction or flexion (usually as a result of weakness of the deltoid, trapezius and serratus anterior muscles). Biomechanically, this instability impairs functional scapular movements in relation to the thorax (what is called altered scapulothoracic kinematics).

As a result of this condition, which is characterized by weakness of the shoulder girdle, chain reactions are created that result in excessive movement in the pelvis and lower back. These attendant movements occur mainly when activating the arm against resistance. The characteristic movement is visible in forward movement of the pelvis when the arms are raised and loads are transferred to the lower back vertebrae (Fig. 6.9).

In this condition, the impaired postural organization in the sagittal plane does not allow the abdominal muscles to stabilize the pelvis and lower back so that they can serve as a base from which arm movements originate, and the result is visible in inefficient movement with cumulative loads along the spine. Therefore, it can be stated that in daily functioning, weakness of the shoulder girdle also affects the spine directly and constitutes an indirect risk factor for the development of back problems.

Shoulder impingement syndrome

Shoulder impingement syndrome is characterized by damage to the normal shoulder movement mechanism, usually as the result of a combination of many repetitions of specific movements, high movement speeds and mechanical pressure exerted on the shoulder, especially in extreme movements of the joint (Bak, 1996; Arroyo et al., 1997).

Intensive physical activity can cause several types of impingement brought on by repetitive movements of the shoulder, and the most common form of impingement has been found to be subacromial impingement (SAI) (Thein & Greenfield, 1997). The structures involved in this pathology are the coracoacromial arch (CAA) (Fig. 6.10) as well as the structures that pass through the subacromial space (SAS).

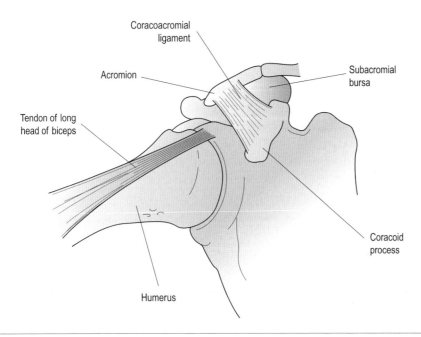

Figure 6.10 Coracoacromial arch (CAA).

The coracoacromial arch encompasses the acromion, the coracoid process and the coracoacromial ligament, which fits into the fibers of the rotator cuff. The unique structure of the coracoacromial arch prevents upper detachment of the humeral head by creating a kind of roof for the subacromial space through which pass the supraspinatus tendon, the subacromial bursa and the upper part of the joint capsule.

A problem in any of the structures of the coracoacromial arch and the subacromial space (SAS) may reduce SAS volume, impinge upon the structures passing through it and as a result, trigger inflammation and pains (Bak, 1996; Arroyo et al., 1997). Under normal conditions, the distance between the borders of the subacromial space in the shoulder is 10 mm, while in a damaged shoulder it is reduced to <6 mm (Thein & Greenfield, 1997).

In many cases characteristic of this condition, the tendon of the supraspinatus muscle, which passes under the scapular coracoid process, is "pinched" by the greater tuberosity of the scapular apex during arm abduction with internal rotation (Warner et al., 1992; Tyler et al., 2000).

The problem begins after repeated friction between the bones and the tendon in the area in which the blood supply to the tendon is inadequate and restricted. As a result of the friction the tendon becomes inflamed, which is evidenced by local swelling and internal hemorrhaging. The local swelling limits range of joint motion and triggers pain during shoulder movements (White & Carmeli, 1999; Ludewig & Cook, 2000).

This inflammatory process usually goes through several stages:

- Slight pains in the shoulder area during rest, which tend to intensify during shoulder movement (mainly against resistance)
- An inflammation in the subscapular bursa. This condition is characterized by pains in the shoulder during flexion or abduction of the arm at 90°
- The sheath over the long head of the biceps brachii may rub against the bicipital groove through which the tendon passes, and may be damaged. Clinical characteristics include prolonged chronic pain (White & Carmeli, 1999). In this condition, impingement may cause a sharp reduction in shoulder functioning: loss of flexibility (reduced range of motion), muscle weakness (especially in the abductor muscles) and a lack of joint stability.

Another type of shoulder impingement, called coracohumeral impingement, occurs in the coracohumeral space (CHS) created by the greater tuberosity and the lesser tuberosity. The structures that pass through it are the subscapularis bursa, subscapularis tendon, and subcoracoid bursa (Thein & Greenfield, 1997).

As noted, shoulder impingement syndrome is prevalent mainly under conditions of physical activity that entail loading on the shoulder girdle. Following are examples of such cases:

1. Swimming-induced impingement syndrome
   Physical impairments in swimming are relatively few, thanks to the lack of vertical load on joints and freedom from having to bear weight. Nevertheless, injuries to the shoulder joint result quite commonly from a combination of repetitive movements and water resistance.

Crawl (freestyle) swimmers are especially sensitive because of the complex movement against resistance that the stroke requires and the broad ranges of motion by the many joints connected to the shoulder girdle. The crawl is the most commonly used stroke in practice. Professional swimmers work out 10–20 h/week, and a session of several kilometers can include thousands of crawl stroke movements. Over the period of 1 year of training, swimmers perform several hundreds of thousands of such movements with each arm. These multiple repetitions over a few years of training, as well as the muscle imbalance that develops around the shoulder, are the main cause leading to the development of impingement syndrome. It is the combination of overload and overuse that causes repetitive injuries in training (Bak, 1996; Bak & Faunl, 1997).

Aside from the frequency of repetitive movements, one of the reasons for the high prevalence of impingement syndrome among crawl swimmers is that the movement used to advance in the water combines medial rotation with arm abduction, performed against strong water resistance (Fig. 6.11). Kinesiologically speaking, this movement combination is problematic because the structural dictates of the shoulder joint require lateral rotation when performing arm abduction beyond a range of 120°, and the rotational movement in the crawl stroke is medial (see Ch. 2).

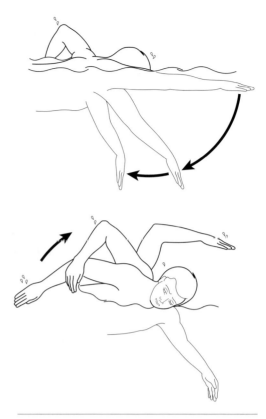

Figure 6.11 Trajectory of arm movements for advancing in water using the crawl stroke.

2. Tennis-induced impingement syndrome

The shoulder area of tennis players must withstand exceptional physical demands, which is why it is subject to injuries. Tennis is a game whose special characteristics require adaptation by the skeletomuscular system. High demands are made on the various joints connected to the shoulder as it tries to attain ranges of motion and speeds combined with rapid transitions from states of acceleration to braking with changes of direction. When the ball hits the racket the shoulder girdle receives a large load by way of the more distal joints (wrist, forearm, and elbow), which are required to function at high speeds and to absorb large loads.

In terms of muscle functioning, as in other sports demanding throwing and pitching movements, tennis encourages the over-development of muscles that rotate inwardly for the serving motion. This creates a muscular imbalance on the dominant side that may trigger the impingement syndrome because of overload in the shoulder area (Schmitt & Snyder, 1999).

3. Vulnerability to shoulder girdle injuries in the gym

   During workouts in the gym, the shoulder girdle is exposed to special forces and loads. To reduce the risk of damage during activity, several kinesiological characteristics should be kept in mind, especially in regard to scapular kinematics.

   Imbalance in scapular position may indirectly damage general shoulder joint stability (Kibler et al., 2002). The scapular muscles help to control scapulohumeral rhythm, which provides optimal contact between the humeral head and the glenoid cavity during abduction. The muscles work synergetically as a force couple (FC), that is, they work with parallel forces in opposite directions to create rotational force on the scapula (McQuade et al., 1998).

   Among the FCs, the relative forces of the trapezius and the serratus anterior are especially prominent. Cooperation between these muscles creates a smooth movement in arm abduction and facilitates dynamic stability of the glenohumeral joint. When the muscles work as a force couple in concentric contraction during arm abduction, they also allow lateral rotation of the scapula, and when they work in eccentric contraction in adduction, they facilitate medial rotation of the scapula.

The following survey reviews several kinesiological aspects stressing the importance of this cooperation for scapular functioning to maintain shoulder stability during arm abduction:

- During the first 90–100° of arm abduction, the center of the scapular rotational axis is located at the base of the scapular spine (Fig. 6.12A). As abduction continues beyond 100°, the center of the scapular rotational axis gradually moves to the acromioclavicular joint (Fig. 6.12B)

- As can be seen in Figure 6.12A, in arm abduction up to 100°, the fibers of the upper trapezius muscle create upward rotation at the scapular apex. At the same time, the serratus anterior pulls the lower corner of the scapula forward and sideways. These two muscles work in tandem to create external rotation of the scapula around an axis located at the base of the scapular spine

- As can be seen in Figure 6.12B, when the arm is raised beyond 100°, the rotational axis of the scapula moves to the acromioclavicular joint. At this stage, the lower fibers of the trapezius become more active as the serratus anterior moves the lower angle (of the scapula) laterally. Normal synergetic cooperation of the muscles allows the humeral head to remain within the joint (the glenoid cavity) while raising the arm.

In light of the above, it is clear that the scapulae play an important role in maintaining dynamic stability of the shoulder joint. Thus, a change in normal scapular position upsets this balancing mechanism, changes the movement axis of the shoulder and creates an imbalance in the forces that are supposed to keep the joint steady (Kibler, 1998; Tyler et al., 2000). In terms of working out in the gym, special caution must be taken, especially when performing strength-building exercises against resistance that place loads on the shoulder girdle.

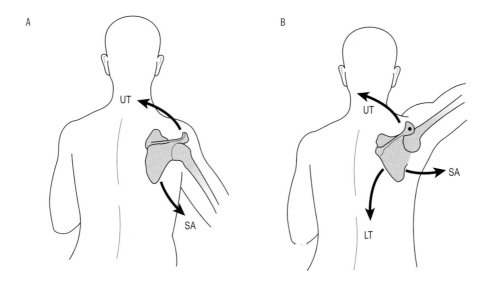

Figure 6.12 Scapular movement with arm raised (A) up to 100° and (B) beyond 100°.

Hyperkinesis and lack of stability in the shoulder girdle

The general ranges of motion in the shoulder are a composite of the sum of the partial movements in the joints connected to it. Viewed in this way, large ranges of motion are made possible by the cooperation of several joints (what is called axillary articulation). The clavicle rotates in relation to the sternum, the scapula rotates in relation to the clavicle, and the humerus moves in relation to the scapula. Moreover, the scapula as a whole creates broad scale rotational movement in relation to the thorax. While this complex structure facilitates very broad ranges of movement, it also makes the task of maintaining stability more difficult.

Lack of stability in the shoulder refers to a large variety of problems characterized by a disruption of the balance of forces that stabilize the shoulder girdle as a whole, and especially the shoulder joint. In addition to the passive structures that stabilize the shoulder, such as the capsule and ligaments, a balance of muscle strength helps to stabilize the joint in dynamic situations (Schmitt & Snyder-Mackler, 1999). These muscles help to maintain the placement of the humeral head within the glenoid cavity and they allow the shoulder joint to remain at the center of the rotational axis of the scapula at all times. When this stabilizing mechanism is impaired, the result is instability, and the humeral head tends to slip partially or fully outside the joint surface of the scapula (Lippitt & Matsen, 1993).

Shoulder instability is manifested as a shifting of the humeral head in one or more directions. The movement limitation is classified according to the extent of slippage and the direction of the deviation (anterior or posterior):

- Anterior instability is the most common condition in cases of shoulder joint instability. Biomechanically, injuries that cause anterior instability usually occur when the shoulder joint is in its weakest position, with the arm in abduction and outward rotation

- Posterior instability, especially trauma-induced posterior dislocation, is less common. Posterior dislocation disrupts the balance between the muscles performing abduction and external rotation of the arm, and those performing adduction and internal rotation. The forces of internal rotation with adduction are stronger, thus exposing the humeral head to posterior dislocation
- Multidirectional instability is usually not caused by acute dislocation but rather as a result of laxity of the passive stabilizing structures (capsule, ligaments) and as the result of weakness of the rotator cuff muscles. These conditions cause hyperflexibility, which in many cases is observable in other joints as well (Warner et al., 1990).

Injuries related to shoulder joint instability are especially apt to occur during physical activity entailing sharp movements, speed and a large range of motion around the joint, as in basketball, volleyball, tennis, golf, and other sports.

The two most common injuries are:

- *Subluxation* – In this condition, the humeral head slips only partially outside the joint boundaries and may return to its place afterwards. This problem is not triggered by trauma and is characterized mainly by conditions of laxity (Taylor & Arciero, 1997)
- *Dislocation* – In this condition, there is complete dislocation, as the entire humeral head is dislodged from the joint cavity. In the first few times, the dislocation is usually associated with strong trauma, but afterwards full dislocation may also result from regular movements. After the initial dislocation, the frequency of subsequent dislocations is high.

Based on the above, the two most common causes of shoulder joint instability are:

1. Trauma that affects the stabilizing structures such as ligaments or the capsule, resulting in dislocation. Common causes of this type of problem are falling, direct blows to the shoulder or strong force applied to the shoulder when the arm is tensed.
2. Laxity and weakness of the passive and active tissues (without previous damage).

Adapted movement for conditions of shoulder instability should be based on a comprehensive orthopedic diagnosis to determine the type of injury. The diagnosis will make it possible to determine not only the type of proper exercise but also which movements are contraindicated and should be avoided. The main emphases in exercise therapy are on a very gradual strengthening of the stabilizing muscles using several types of contractions. During the initial stages of rehabilitation, the emphasis is placed on isometric contraction that facilitates strengthening processes without movement in the joint. At later stages the exercises begin with the arm in a position of adduction, then flexion, and gradually work up to strengthening the arm in abduction. Exercises for improving shoulder girdle stability appear in detail later in this chapter.

Functional rigidity of the shoulder girdle

Rigidity in the shoulder sharply decreases range of motion in one or more of the joints connected to the shoulder girdle. Movement limitations in this area can originate from any of a number of causes, such as rigidity due to faulty posture patterns (kyphosis), emotional problems (heightened muscle tone resulting from stress), traumatic damage (sport injuries) and physiological problems such as osteoarthritis.

The most common causes of functional rigidity in the shoulder are:

1. Postural disorders characterized by rounded back and excessive protrusion of the thoracic vertebrae. In most cases, these conditions cause a drawing forward of the shoulders and a shortening of the chest muscles (pectoralis major/pectoralis minor). The result is general rigidity of the shoulder, which is characterized by a postural stance in which the arms are rotated inward and the scapulae are in protraction (see Ch. 3).

   Movement treatment of these conditions combines exercises to improve ranges of motion for the muscles mentioned above, with exercises for moving all the joints connected to the shoulder girdle, including the joints between the sternum and the ribs (sternocostal joints) and the ribs and the vertebrae (costovertebral joints) (Kisner & Colby, 1985).

2. Functional rigidity caused by osteoarthritis. Osteoarthritis is a chronic disease that usually involves the peripheral joints (arms and legs) and causes a progressive acceleration of attritional processes. As a result, degenerative changes may occur in the skeletal system as well as in joint cartilage. These changes trigger an inflammatory reaction which later develops chronic pains around the affected joint.

   Movement problems in the shoulder joint as a result of osteoarthritis may be traceable to a number of causes, such as infection, damage to the immune system or genetic-hereditary factors. Common movement characteristics of this condition are:

   - Sensitivity and pains that intensify during physical activity
   - A decrease in ranges of motion and a functional rigidity that tends to worsen over time
   - Development of deformations in the affected joint resulting from the destruction of cartilage and a weakening of soft tissues such as muscles and ligaments.

Movement treatment for shoulder joint problems caused by osteoarthritis:

In addition to medicative intervention, exercise therapy is very important for preserving range of motion and strengthening the stabilizing muscles. At the same time, because of the progressive nature of the problem, movement treatment in these cases should be based on a comprehensive medical diagnosis and should be carried out by a certified therapist, as overload may accelerate the processes of joint attrition.

3. Functional rigidity caused by frozen shoulder

   Frozen shoulder is manifested by rigidity and limitations in shoulder movement accompanied by pain. Such a condition may have any number of causes, such as traumatic injuries (dislocation, fracture, torn muscle), spinal problems, neurological problems, and even heart disease, diabetes or thyroid dysfunction, among others (Sandor & Brone, 2000). As symptoms may indicate several possibilities, it is often difficult to diagnose the source of the problem.

   During its initial stages, there is sensitivity in the joint, followed by slight pain that tends to intensify during certain movements or in physical positions that involve weight bearing (such as lying on the problematic side). Over time, an inflammation develops in the soft tissues (passive and active) both in and around the shoulder joint, creating functional weakness and severe rigidity that limit the range of motion and impair optimal functioning of the shoulder during activities of daily living (ADL). In the movement treatment of frozen shoulder the emphasis is on using adapted physical activity as part of the array of treatments–often also including medication–available to medical personnel. At the same time, therapeutic exercise to improve range of motion is important from the time the problem first begins to appear.

   In movement treatment, ways must be found to move the joint in conditions or at movement angles that do not engender pain. Adapted exercises integrate variations of passive and active movements in closed and open kinematic chains. Movements that are especially sensitive to pain usually include arm abduction and lateral rotation against resistance, and in treatment (as in ADL), it is important to find ways to circumvent them (e.g., using a ladder in order to bring down an object from above head level). Exercises and theoretical principles for building an exercise program to improve shoulder girdle kinesis appear later in this chapter.

Adapted physical activity for functional disorders of the shoulder joint and shoulder girdle

Effective treatment to improve shoulder girdle kinesis should be based on a full functional evaluation of all the factors affecting joint movements. To this end, therapists must understand the complexity of the functional chain affecting the shoulder girdle. Kinesiologically speaking, it can be said that "the body takes movement to where it is most comfortable". In other words, there is a tendency to circumvent a limitation in a given joint by using a chain reaction and transferring the movement to neighboring joints.

As a result, limitations of movement ranges in a given area can cause hyperkinesis in another area. This kinesiological aspect takes on a variety of patterns in the shoulder girdle. The following are examples of common chain reactions resulting from disorders in shoulder functioning:

1. When flexing arms (against resistance), weakness of the muscles stabilizing the shoulder girdle creates a reaction of forward movement of the pelvis and hyperkinesis of the lower back vertebrae (see Fig. 6.9).

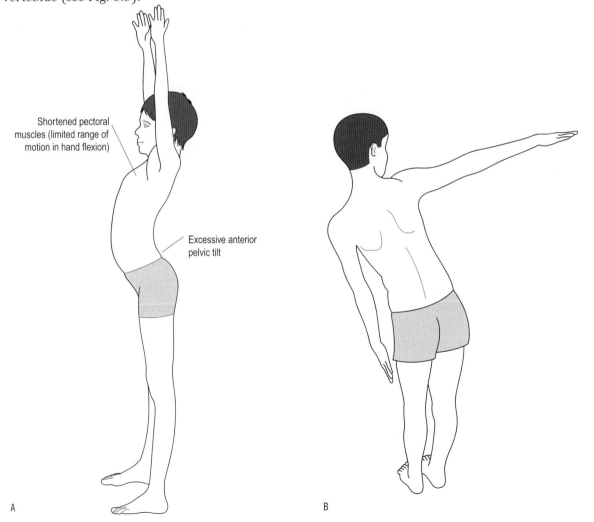

Shortened pectoral muscles (limited range of motion in hand flexion)

Excessive anterior pelvic tilt

A

B

Figure 6.13 Chain reactions in the pelvis and lower back as a result of functional disorders of the shoulder. (A) Excessive forward movement of the pelvis as a chain reaction to shortened pectoral muscles when raising arms. (B) Accompanying movements in the pelvic and back areas with functional rigidity of the shoulder during arm abduction.

2. When performing various movements requiring the raising of arms above head level, functional rigidity of the shoulder creates chain reactions of anterior pelvic tilt (APT) and accompanying movements in the lower back vertebrae (Fig. 6.13).

3. Functional shortening of pectoralis minor causes scapular protraction and draws the shoulders forward. This condition creates a kyphotic position of the upper back, and heightens muscular tension in the area of the cervical and lumbar spine (see Ch. 3).

These and many other examples indicate the importance of accurate diagnosis of the source of the problem as a basis for effective treatment of faulty movement patterns. The next section presents examples of exercises intended to improve various shoulder girdle functions impaired by the disorders described in this chapter.

Exercises for general functional improvement of scapular mobility in relation to the thorax (scapulothoracic kinesis)

Successful treatment to improve shoulder girdle movement is based on a comprehensive diagnosis of all postural patterns (see also Ch. 7). In most cases general improvement of postural patterns is an essential part of treating the scapulae.

Movement treatment to improve scapular functioning can employ closed or open kinematic chain exercises.

Closed kinematic chain exercises

These exercises are an effective way to improve the functioning of muscles that work on the scapulae, making use of a wall or the ground for support while activating the scapula in all movement possibilities (Fig. 6.14A–G). The starting positions may contribute to improving movement patterns and stimulate muscle contraction in a variety of functional angles.

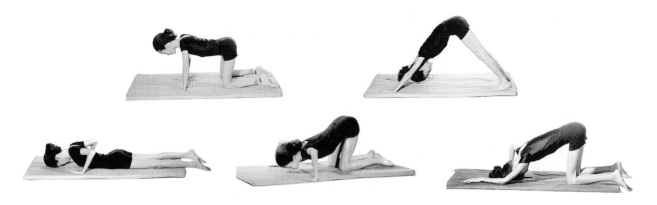

Figure 6.14 Examples of starting positions adapted for moving the shoulder girdle in a closed kinematic chain (hands fixed on the ground). (See also: free movement within a structured framework in Ch. 9.)

Open kinematic chain exercises

These exercises allow patients to progress to complex movements in larger ranges of motion around the shoulder joint (Fig. 6.15).

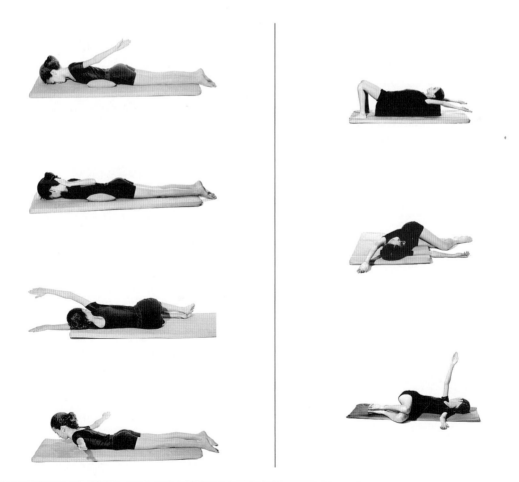

Figure 6.15 Examples of starting positions adapted to move the shoulder girdle in an open kinematic chain.

The following exercises are intended for overall improvement of scapulothoracic mobility.

These exercises may also be suitable for cases of frozen shoulder. Chapter 8 presents additional exercises intended to lengthen pectoral muscles and they may also be suitable for improving scapulothoracic mobility.

1. *Standing*: rotation movements inward and outward as an indirect means of making the scapula perform protraction–retraction. Performing the movements unilaterally (one arm) and bilaterally (both arms simultaneously).

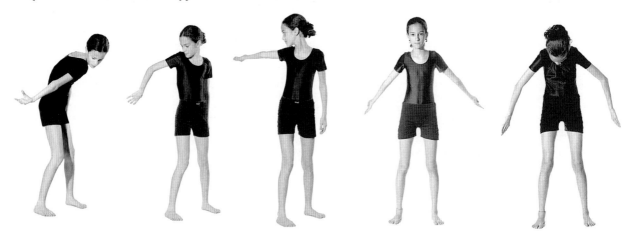

2. *Lying face down*: forehead or cheek on the floor, fingers interlaced above the pelvis: raising hands upwards with fingers interlaced and bringing scapulae closer together.

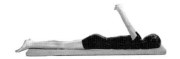

3. *Lying face down*: one arm straight ahead, the opposite knee flexed: alternating arm and leg positions as if "crawling in place". This emphasizes scapular mobility on the frontal plane.

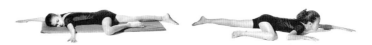

4. *Standing on hands and knees*: moving one arm up, down and in various directions.

   The movement can be performed in various starting positions (paying attention to arm and leg position).

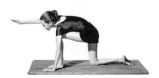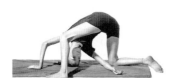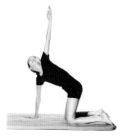

5. *Sitting cross-legged*: moving arms in various directions: up, down and back.

   Interlacing hands behind the back encourages scapular adduction.

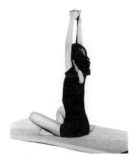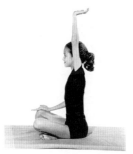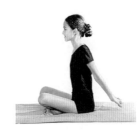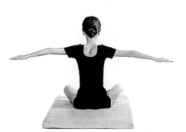

6. *Lying on side, knees bent to the chest, arms straight to the side at face level*: creating circular movements (with upper arm) around the body, moving the head in the same direction.

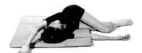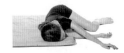

7. *Lying on a bench or treatment bed, knees bent*: holding a stick with both hands under the bench, lowering knees from side to side until there is a feeling of lengthening in the chest muscles.

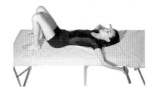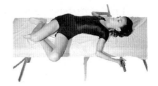

8. *Lying on back*: stretching arms backwards, dorsiflexing the feet and lowering arms to the sides along the body.

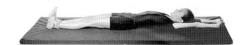

9. *Lying on bench, knees bent*, hands holding a stick under the bench: straightening and stretching arms, and flexing them until scapulae are brought towards each other. In this position, lowering knees from side to side.

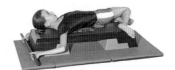
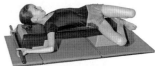

10. *Standing*: holding a stick behind the back.

    • On exhalation – bending the torso forward with knees bent, bringing the chin to the sternum, and leading the stick upward
    • On inhalation – rising with long back.

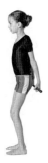
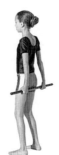
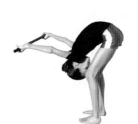
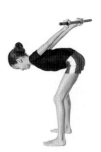

11. *Standing one leg forward*: holding a stick behind the back.

    • On exhalation – bending the torso forward with knees bent, and leading the stick upward
    • On inhalation – rising with long back.

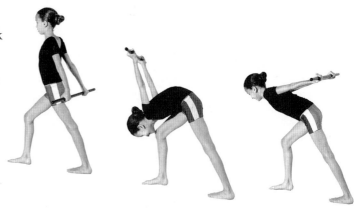

12. *Sitting on a chair*: holding a stick slightly beyond shoulder width.

- Raising the stick and lowering it to scapula height
- Rotational (twisting) movements of the torso from side to side (knees facing straight forward).

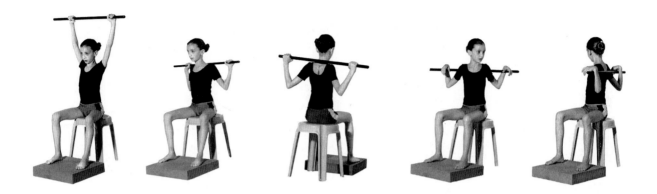

Movement treatment for instability in the shoulder girdle

The main aim of the following exercises is to improve shoulder girdle stability. It is important to promote dynamic stability of the shoulder joint by means of exercises that strengthen all of the muscles ensheathing it, and especially the rotator cuff muscles that stabilize the humeral head in the glenoid cavity.

Exercises 1–4 make use of an elastic fitness band that provides resistance in various kinds of contraction. It is possible to attach the band to a ladder or wall at various heights.

1. Standing – elbow flexed 90° and held close to the body, hand holding the band: concentric and eccentric contraction of the muscles rotating the arm outward by stretching the band and slowly returning to the starting position.

    The elbow is held close to the trunk throughout the range of motion.

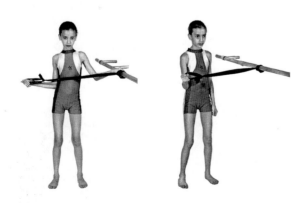

2. Standing – holding the band at waist level, elbow flexed to 90° and held close to the body: stretching the band while concentrically and eccentrically contracting the muscles that rotate the arm inward.

   The movement can be performed unilaterally (one arm) or bilaterally (two arms using two bands simultaneously).

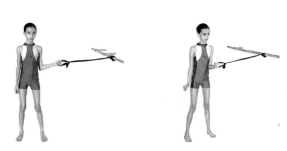

3. Standing – stretching the band while abducting arm to 90° and returning it slowly to starting position (concentric and eccentric contraction of arm abductor muscles).

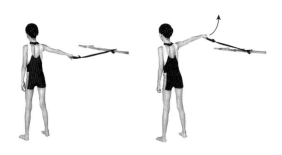

4. Standing – or sitting – holding the band at shoulder level: stretching the band by contracting the arm adductor muscles.

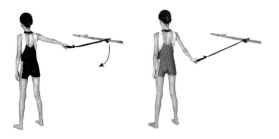

5. Standing – stretching the band while extending the arm backwards, and returning it slowly to starting position (concentric and eccentric contraction of arm extensor muscles).

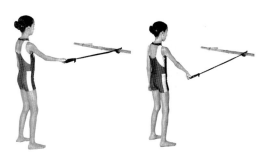

6. Standing on hands and knees – lowering forehead to the floor and performing isometric contraction by pushing hands downward.

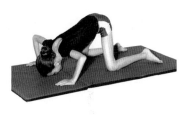

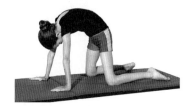

7. Lying face down, hands placed under shoulders, elbows facing upward and close to body – pushing against the floor and raising the trunk slightly while adducting and lowering scapulae.

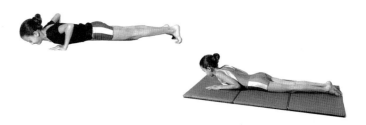

8. Lying face down (a pillow can be placed under the abdomen), forehead to the floor and arms spread to the sides – raising arms in various ways while adducting the scapulae towards one another.

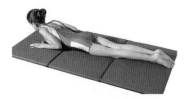 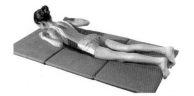 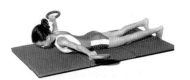

9. Standing – or sitting – abducting arms to 90° while adducting the scapulae towards one another (a small hand weight can be held during the exercise).

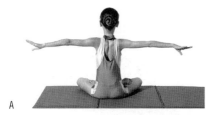

A

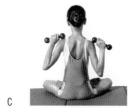

C

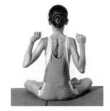

B

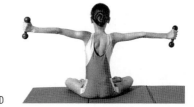

D

Exercises to strengthen the serratus anterior muscle in cases of wing scapulae

In most cases of wing scapulae, it is helpful to strengthen the serratus anterior muscle separately as a means of tightening the scapulae to the thorax. This is accomplished by the following exercises:

1. Exercises using a physiotherapy ball.
   - Standing on hands and knees over the ball: transferring body weight to hands while breaking knee–ground contact; pushing against the floor while extending elbows until upper back is rounded

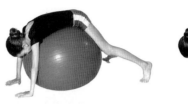 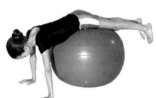

   - Placing lower legs on the ball: pushing against the floor with straight arms in order to abduct scapulae from one another

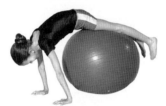 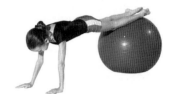

   - Standing on hands and knees, arms resting on ball: breaking knee–ground contact while pressing on the ball and rounding the upper back (upward).

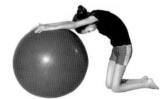

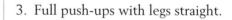

2. Push-ups, knees on floor: emphasizing the push against the floor until full scapular abduction is attained.

3. Full push-ups with legs straight.

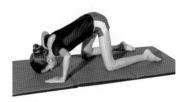 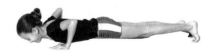

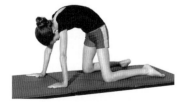 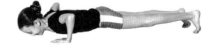

4. Push-ups, elbows straight: on exhalation, pushing against the floor while holding in the abdomen and rounding the upper back.

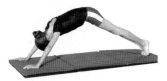

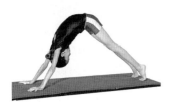

5. Push-ups with legs on bench or step: on exhalation, holding in the abdomen and pushing the chest up until scapulae are abducted from one another.

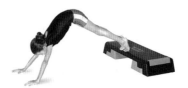

6. Push-ups on a step: ascending and descending the step hand after hand maintaining straightened elbows.

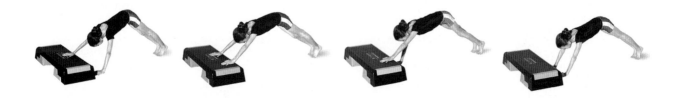

7. Lying on back, feet on floor near pelvis, holding hand weights of 3–5 kg: pushing the weights up with arms straight.

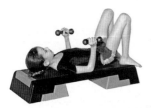

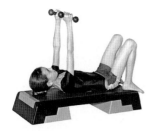

8. Holding a stick with an elastic fitness band tied to both ends: lying on back with feet on floor and band under scapulae, pushing the stick upward with straight elbows.

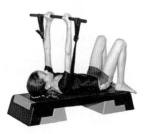

9. Standing or lying on back, holding the band with both hands, band on scapular area: on exhalation, stretching the band forward, elbows straight.

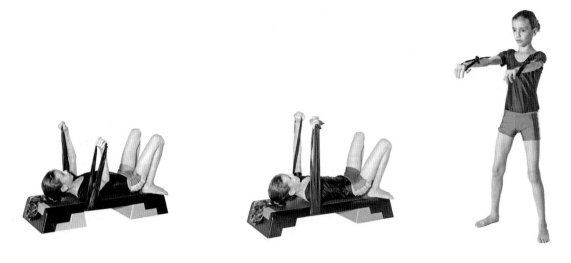

10. One leg forward, facing wall, hands placed on wall at shoulder height: on exhalation, pushing the wall with elbows straight while rounding the upper back and abducting the scapulae.

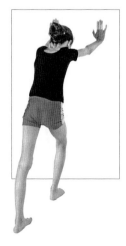 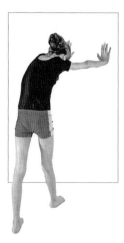

Emphases in adapted movement treatment to improve functionality in cases of shoulder impingement syndrome

At all stages of a rehabilitation program for shoulder impingement syndrome, it is recommended to avoid entering the pain cycle and to instruct patients not to perform exercises on their own when they are in pain. The reason is that impingement-induced pain may trigger a series of changes that is manifest in muscle inhibition, which alters the scapulohumeral rhythm and creates muscular imbalance around the shoulder. This condition may reduce the subacromial space (SAS), increase stresses activated on it and aggravate the impingement (Hess, 2000; Wilk et al., 2002).

A gradual program for treating shoulder injuries is usually divided into stages:

1. In the acute stage, which entails pain, it is important to avoid pain-inducing actions. The aim of this stage is to reduce pain by rest, and when necessary, by the use of anti-inflammatory medications (Arroyo, 1997; Wilk et al., 2002).
2. It is recommended to gradually begin to restore normative ranges of motion in the shoulder using passive and active movements and muscle stretches.
3. Exercises for gradually strengthening the shoulder girdle can be individually adapted to the characteristics of the specific problem, with extreme caution taken not to apply excess loads that might induce pain.

Many of the exercises described in this chapter may also be suitable to the movement treatment of shoulder impingement syndrome, but any exercise program for this problem should be performed under medical supervision only.

Exercises for general strengthening of the shoulder girdle

The main objective of the following exercises is to strengthen the shoulder girdle through full ranges of movements on all planes. The following exercises utilize a number of auxiliary aids.

1. Sitting on a chair – arms up – hands holding a rubber fitness band at shoulder width. Stretching the rubber band downward and upward while concentrically and eccentrically contracting the muscles that adduct the arms.

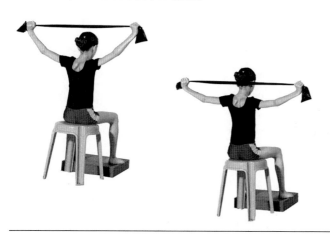

2. Lying face down – arms straight ahead – holding the rubber fitness band at shoulder width.

   - Stretching the band while adducting and abducting the arms.

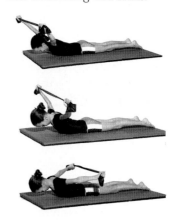

3. Lying face down. Holding a stick behind the back (at pelvic width). (The stick should be held downwards so that the arms are turned outward.)

   - On exhalation – raising the torso while adducting the scapulae
   - During the movement it is possible to create isometric contraction of the adductor muscles (by "pressing" the stick towards the center) or of the abductors (by "stretching" the stick towards the sides).

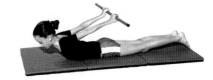

4. Lying face down – arms straight ahead. Connecting two long rubber fitness bands cross-wise (using looped connections on the diagonal – right foot to left hand, and left foot to right hand).

   - On inhalation lift legs, torso and arms upward
   - On exhalation – lower them forward

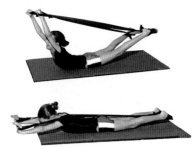

   - Performing movements of adduction and abduction while concentrically and eccentrically contracting the shoulder abductors.

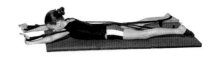

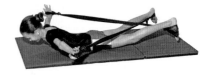

5. Lying face down on a mat or step – arms straight forward and holding a stick.

   - Lifting the stick with arms straight
   - Lifting the stick up and then leading it towards the scapulae while bending the elbows
   - Tying a rope to the center of the stick and pulling at the rope by the therapist: allows the patient to create resistance adjusted to the working muscles.

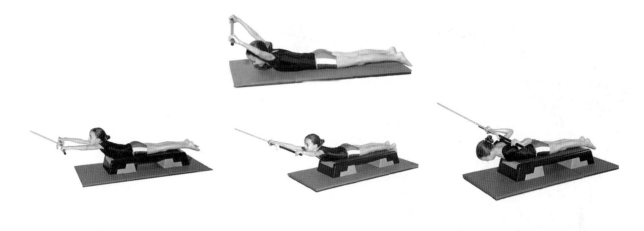

6. Lying on the back on a step, knees bent, feet close to pelvis.

   - Holding a stick at shoulder width. Rope tied to the stick for providing resistance adjusted to the working muscles
   - Flexing and extending the arms against resistance
   - Changing the position of the therapist while using the tied stick will make it possible to provide resistance to the shoulder flexor and extensor muscles.

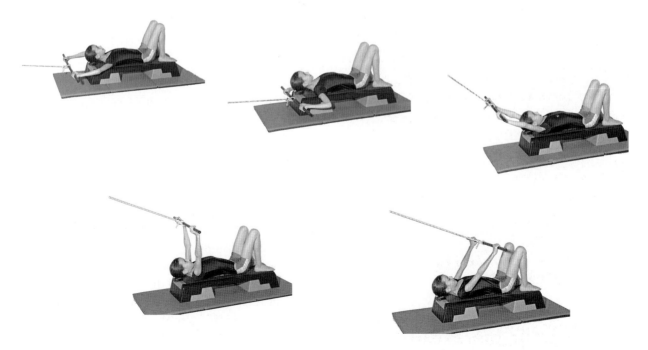

CHAPTER 7

Principles for a comprehensive diagnosis of postural disorders

Many theories have been published to "explain" why and how physical disorders and pathologies develop. Underlying any individual problem is usually one true "scenario" that triggered development of the disorder. This scenario is not always evident, and in most cases, its roots are quite complex. This makes the diagnostician's job complex, and underscores the need to avoid hasty decisions which might lead to wrong conclusions.

In his book *Living, Loving and Learning,* Leo Buscaglia (1982) describes the prevailing diagnostic approach to special children. "Our way of looking at children is interesting. The speech therapist

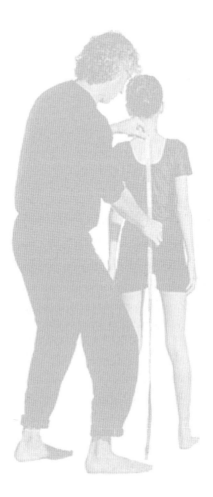

sees the child as a case of stuttering or of speech hindrance, the occupational therapist sees the child as a motor problem, the school psychologist sees the child as a learning or emotional problem, the physiotherapist sees the same child as an array of movement problems, and the neurologist uncovers behavioral responses. Then there are the parents who try to see their child as a whole entity but it does not take us long to convince them that there is no such thing, and then they lose their comprehensive view of their child's latent abilities, and in their eyes, he or she becomes a 'problem child'."

All of these "experts" see only what they have been trained to consider as the crux of the problem, and the truth is that what they see actually exists in that child. But a child is much more than a symptom, so much so that the essence, the most important piece of the puzzle, may be completely hidden from view.

In this vein, it is worth remembering Maslov's statement that if the only tool one has is a hammer, one will tend to treat all things like a nail. Therefore, when viewing children, therapists must see them as they are, as many things – some overt, others covert – and many "tools" are necessary for working with them. This is the approach that should be applied to both diagnosis and treatment.

Questionnaire for parents

The Little Prince returned to the fox. "Goodbye to you", he said when the time of departure arrived. "Go in good health", replied the fox. "Here is my secret and it is very simple: Do not look at things only in the heart, because the important thing is really hidden from view". "Everything important is hidden from view", repeated the Little Prince so that it would be engraved in his heart (Antoine de Saint-Exupéry).

Many therapists who work with children have become more mellow over the years with regard to the influence they exert on the lives of the children they treat. They learn that success in their work with children depends first and foremost on the quality of their ties with the parents and the extent of the parents' support for the treatment.

Parental motivation is a moving force for change that can and should be utilized for the good of the children who require treatment. The therapist's challenge in addressing children's problems is how to harness this motivation to yield cooperative work.

Parents are the most important source of information about their children's development and environment, information that is essential to understand the child's personality and problems.

The aim at this stage of diagnosis is to obtain general information from the parents about their children. This information forms a basis for deciding what to examine in the coming diagnostic stages. The most important points of reference have been selected from the many questions that parents should be asked at this stage (Appendix 1) (Solberg, 1998a):

- The background of the problem and the reason for seeking treatment
- The course of pregnancy and birth
- The child's general development from birth
- Motor development – did the child go through all the developmental stages (turning over, crawling, sitting, standing, walking, running) within the normal time range
- Present motor functioning – any limitations or functional difficulties in daily life
- Cognitive functioning (comprehension)
- Affective functioning – fears, coping with difficulties, frustration threshold, self-esteem, expression of emotions
- Behavioral functioning
- Social status and communication with other children
- Other problems, illnesses, use of medications, allergies, etc.

Diagnosing posture

One of the most pervasive problems facing therapists working with children with postural disorders arises from the difficulty of using tests and measurements that allow reliable monitoring of the progress and results of treatment. Without these periodic tests, therapists are hard pressed to determine what effect, if any, their treatment has actually had on the children's condition, and as a result, they base their work more on intuition and less on objective, reliable data. The posture evaluation presented in this chapter is based on a broad array of data which, if properly analyzed, will provide an adequately reliable diagnosis of a child's condition.

In diagnosing posture, information can be gathered in a number of ways:

- Subjective evaluation by observing the standing individual from the side, front and back
- Anthropometric measurements that provide objective information about body proportions such as length of the lower extremities, scapula height, etc
- Functional muscle testing and ranges of joint motion
- X-rays.

The posture examination form presented in this chapter is intended for professionals, and its purpose is to help therapists to conduct their tests in a logical order and to record their findings concisely. The information obtained from these tests is usually sufficient, but in certain cases other tests may have to be added or alterations made to existing ones.

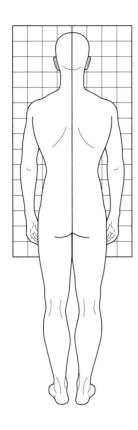

Posture examination form

Date:
Name:
Surname:
Gender: M / F
Date of birth:

General Examination:

a. Posterior view

1. Achilles tendon and feet: Right _____   Left _____
2. Knees (genu varum/genu valgum) _____
3. Pelvic balance (posterior/superior iliac spine) _____
4. Scapulae (height, distance from spine, rotation) _____
5. Shoulder line _____
6. Neck _____
7. Symmetry of fat folds (pelvis, waist, neck) _____
8. Spinal column (scoliosis) _____

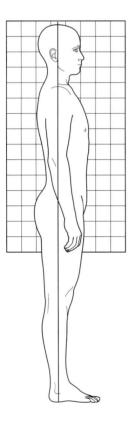

b. Lateral view

1. Feet arches _____
2. Knees (hyperextension) _____
3. Pelvis (posterior/anterior tilt) _____
4. Spinal curves (kyphosis/lordosis/flat back) _____
5. Shoulder position _____
6. Head position (cervical lordosis) _____

c. Anterior view

1. Feet _____
2. Knees _____
3. Pelvis (anterior superior iliac spine) _____
4. Shoulders height _____
5. Neck/Head _____

Functional tests (*Figs 7.1–7.13*)

1. Length of spinal column (C7–S1) _____
   Standing: _____ Forward bending: _____
2. General flexibility test: _____
   Legs straight _____
   Forward bending with knees bent _____
3. Hamstrings flexibility (SLR):   Right _____ Left _____
4. Quadratus lumborum flexibility _____
5. Thomas Test for iliopsoas flexibility: Right _____ Left _____
6. Abdominal muscle strength _____
7. Ability to flatten lower back to floor (lying supine) _____
8. Range of shoulder motion: Right _____ Left _____
9. Length of lower extremities: Right _____ Left _____
10. Back muscle strength: Cervical erectors _____
    Erector spinae _____
    Scapulae adductors _____
11. Shoulder girdle strength:
    Abduction: Right _____ Left _____
    Adduction: Right _____ Left _____
    Flexion: Right _____ Left _____
    Extension: Right _____ Left _____
12. Static balance: Right leg _____ Left leg _____
13. Dynamic balance: _____
14. Forward walking (general evaluation – broad/narrow support base, movement balance, movement flow, coordination) _____

_____
_____

X-rays, medical documents and previous diagnoses:

_____
_____

General evaluation:

_____
_____

Recommended treatment (indications/contraindications):

_____
_____

Figure 7.1 Observation from back and front to identify postural disorders on the coronal (frontal) plane.

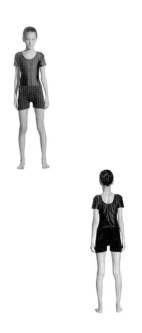

Figure 7.2 Observation from the side to identify postural disorders on the sagittal plane.

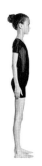

Figure 7.3 Examination of spinal length standing and bent forward.

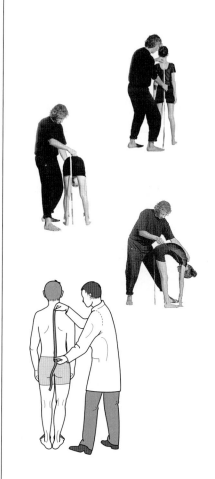

Figure 7.4 General flexibility test, with legs straight and with bent knees.

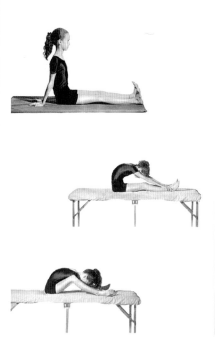

Figure 7.5 Test of straight leg raising (hamstring muscle flexibility).

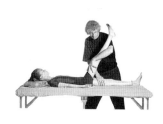

Figure 7.6 Subjective test to evaluate quadratus lumborum flexibility.

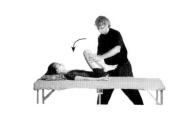
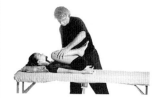

Figure 7.7 Thomas Test to check iliopsoas muscle.

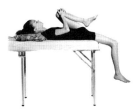

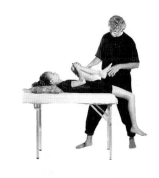

Figure 7.9 Examination of lower extremity length.

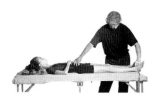

Figure 7.13 Ways to evaluate range of motion in the shoulder girdle.

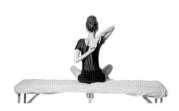

Figure 7.10 Test of cervical erector strength.

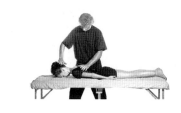

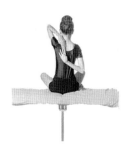

Figure 7.11 Test of erector spinae strength.

Figure 7.8 Test of abdominal muscle strength.

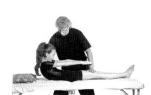

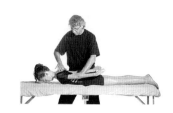

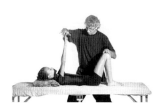

Figure 7.12 Test of scapulae adductor strength (shoulder extensors).

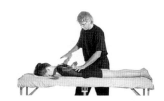

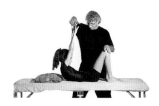

Psychomotor diagnosis

One of the important skills diagnosticians must have is the ability to get to know the child and respond to his condition; they must understand the patterns, systems and processes that brought him to his present state. This stage of psychomotor ability diagnosis helps diagnosticians to become better acquainted with the children they are going to treat so that they can adapt the therapeutic contents and approach to the children's personality and special needs (Solberg, 1998b, 1999). The basic assumption underlying this chapter is that postural disorders, whether arising from emotional or physical sources, also affect children's movement patterns.

The characteristic limitations that children with postural disorders experience – such as muscle weakness, heightened muscle tone, limited ranges of motion or functional asymmetry resulting from incorrect positioning of one or more joints – necessarily affect functions such as balance, coordination, movement precision and strength regulation. Problems in these motor functions may cause other impediments to basic skills such as balanced walking and running and performance of various ball skills. In many cases, these difficulties are characterized by motor clumsiness.

Since movement and motor ability play such an important role in building children's self confidence and self esteem, those suffering from basic functional deficits may experience a loss of self confidence, develop emotional tension, and later become enmeshed in the "vicious cycle" described in Figure 7.14.

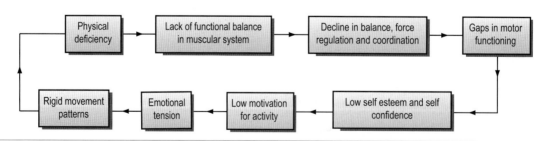

Figure 7.14 Interaction between postural disorders and emotional problems.

In order to ensure effective and correct treatment of the problem, therapists should try to "break" this cycle and build a new one. One of the ways to do this in working with children is through motor activity (Fig. 7.15).

The term "psychomotorics" refers to the interaction of motor and emotional control processes that also include perceptive, cognitive, and emotional components. The term psychomotorics emphasizes the close interrelations between emotional processes and motor phenomena (Hutzler, 1990). The psychomotor approach views movement as a complex phenomenon that integrates feelings and thoughts as well as the body's physiological systems. The aim of psychomotor diagnosis is to add another important facet to overall diagnosis of the children in order to establish a baseline on which to build the therapeutic process (Hutzler, 1990).

Psychomotoric disturbance includes deviant postural patterns, motor clumsiness, impaired muscle tone, movement disorders such as hypo/hyperkinesis, and others. One of the main aims of the examinations is to test children's overall motor ability on the assumption that this multi-faceted ability will allow them to perform a broad array of motor tasks (Solberg, 1998b).

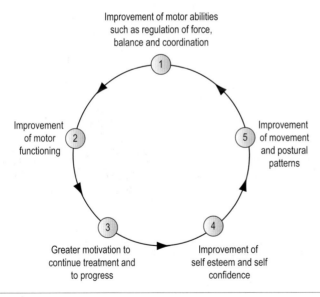

Figure 7.15 Improvement of motor functioning as a means of improving postural patterns.

General guidelines for psychomotor diagnosis

As noted, diagnosis and evaluation are initial milestones of any therapeutic program. The approach proposed in this chapter emphasizes a holistic view of the many components and characteristics comprising patients' personality and abilities, in both the physical and the emotional domains. This model was developed to help therapists to improve their ability to observe, diagnose, process data and build the most appropriate treatment program.

It should be kept in mind that diagnosis is an ongoing dynamic process that offers the opportunity to define a person's current condition as a whole. Therefore, each meeting throughout the treatment process creates a change that confirms or alters the therapist's conclusions. Thus, each meeting renews the diagnostic process.

This chapter will present a number of options for examining each domain in order to allow diagnosticians as much "room to maneuver" as possible in their professional decisions about the type of examination and the level required. This material can also serve as an idea bank to be referenced during the treatment stage as well. The examinations are based on subjective evaluations of each patient according to that patient's functional level, and according to universal measures. While this applied approach is appropriate for therapists working in a clinic, it is not suitable for research that requires more precise objective tests under laboratory conditions.

Because adapting examination techniques to children is a true "art" that diagnosticians should develop, it is important to maintain a great deal of flexibility of thought when diagnosing and to try not to work mechanically according to set schemas.

The evaluation scale presented for summarizing the data is based, as noted, on subjective evaluation using a 5-point scale for evaluating ability in each domain (Table 7.1).

Table 7.1 Posture evaluation scale

EVALUATION	QUALITY OF PERFORMANCE
1	Very weak
2	Weak
3	Moderate
4	Good
5	Very good

Summarizing data in this manner allows therapists to continually monitor children's progress in each domain, and based on their condition, to adapt the "line of action".

The suggested tests have been divided into specific domains that inform therapists about children's functioning on various levels. After defining the subject of each test, the text will provide examples for gathering information in that domain. It is important to keep in mind that the test options have infinite variations, and basing themselves on this material, diagnosticians can utilize their experience to develop additional approaches.

The tests for each domain are presented as follows:

1. Introduction to the test
2. How to perform it
3. Emphases for observation. This section mentions the points to observe closely as the child performs the task. In some cases, reference is made to other domains not directly connected to what is being tested but that give an indication of how the child functions in other spheres as well. As already mentioned, the aim of the diagnosis is to collect as much information about the child as possible, and the guiding principle is to obtain maximum information about all possible domains from each movement task.

It should be kept in mind that performance of certain motor tasks reflects a number of underlying abilities. Experienced diagnosticians observing a child bouncing a basketball, for example, can glean much information about that child's visuomotor coordinative ability, force regulation, timing, movement isolation and movement precision. As to posture, diagnosticians will be especially interested in the array of motor abilities affecting movement and posture patterns such as balance, kinesthesis, force regulation, differentiated movement and coordination.

Main areas of examination in psychomotor diagnosis

Coordination Many daily activity movements require coordination between different body parts, such as arms and legs in walking, or eyes and extremities in ball skills. The right and left cerebral hemispheres function together integratively and cooperatively. The quality of cerebral functioning depends on the functional ability of each side independently, especially on the integration between them by means of pathways that connect the two sides.

Coordination makes movement efficient, flowing and energetically economical. Coordination is reflected in a person's ability to combine a number of movements into a flowing pattern that integrates a number of systems, such as the musculoskeletal and nervous systems with the senses of sight, hearing and kinesthesis.

Impaired coordination between body systems, whether internal or external, indicates a flaw in holistic functioning. The effect of such poor functioning on children with coordinative difficulties is tremendous frustration, because their bodies do not do what they want them to do and they feel that their body control has been undermined. In most cases, such difficulty also has affective ramifications, which are often evidenced in lowered self esteem and self confidence. Children tend to lose their footing because of lack of movement balance, they drop a ball thrown to them in a game, and they find play and activities – which other children consider joyful and natural – to be a source of difficulty.

Normal coordination, which facilitates optimal balance between stability and movement, depends on normal functioning of the nervous system as it receives and analyzes information and then directs implementation of normal movement patterns.

Many postural disorders may develop as a result of coordination problems. Under normal circumstances, the messages carried by the peripheral nerves pick up information from the sensory systems and transmit orders to the skeletal muscles. This fine and precise control is made possible by the continuous feedback of information received from the movement. This information undergoes processing, which creates a pattern of new motor responses (Schmidt, 1988).

Normal postural patterns are possible thanks to control over this process, so that in each movement, some muscles are recruited for activity, while others remain in a relaxed state (movement differentiation). Difficulties here may cause many excess movements, heightened muscle tone and rigid movement patterns. In this case, treatment that focuses only on releasing muscle tone without trying to improve the coordinative problems will not yield good results because it does not deal with the root of the problem.

The aim of diagnosis and its consequent treatment is to identify the source of the difficulty and to alter the situation accordingly. Diagnosticians must be sensitive to children's coordinative functioning so that they can feel when a given task becomes a focus of frustration and stress, and when it imbues children with a feeling of confidence. This explains the importance of diagnosticians' skill in building a graduated 'remedial process' that does not frustrate the children but rather makes them feel confident by giving many opportunities for success.

A number of components (given below) must act integratively to produce the conditions for coordinated movement.

Regulation of force This is reflected in the ability to perform a movement precisely and to adjust the amplitude of force required for its performance. Normal regulation of force allows children to invest the correct amount of energy in terms of the number of motor units that contract in the muscle.

Differentiated movement This affects the ability to activate each body limb separately and effectively while releasing excessive muscle tone in other body limbs. The result is no additional points of tension that do not contribute to movement.

Balance Balance affects the ability to change the base of support freely thus allowing a flowing, smooth transition from one position to the next while maintaining a state of balance.

Kinesthesis This allows children to feel the placement of their body limbs in the environment while controlling a variety of movements with no visual feedback (see Ch. 2).

In light of the above, treating postural problems should link these components together and relate to each of them in the exercises (Fig. 7.16).

The following tests enable information to be obtained on the patient's ability in every one of the aspects shown above.

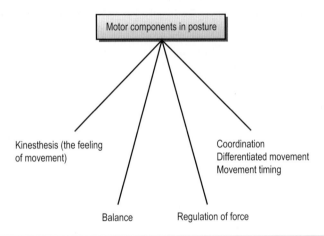

Figure 7.16 Important motor components for maintaining normal posture.

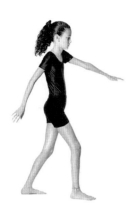

Tests to evaluate coordination and movement timing

1. Step leaps

   Instructions: Standing in a walking position, right leg forward, left arm (opposite) lifted to front and right arm backwards. Leaping and switching arm and leg positions simultaneously and sequentially. Emphases for observation:

   a. Arm–leg coordination in opposing movements
   b. Movement flow – are the leaps sequential or choppy?

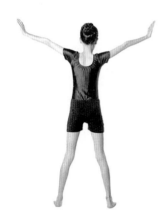

2. Leg-spread leaps

   Instructions: From standing erect with arms beside body – leaping to a spread leg stance while bringing arms up to shoulder height at the same time; then back to starting position without stopping. Emphases for observation:

   a. Arm–leg coordination
   b. Movement flow.

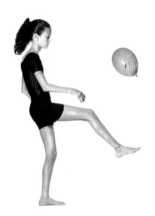

3. Kicking and catching a balloon

   Instructions: Standing – throwing balloon into the air with two hands. As it falls, kicking it and catching it again with both hands. Emphases for observation:

   a. Eye–foot coordination
   b. Correct timing in kicking ball up
   c. Ability to balance body on one foot while kicking
   d. Force regulation in kicking ball up.

Figure 7.17 Tests to evaluate coordination and movement timing.

4. Move ball around body while walking

   Instructions: Walking forward in a straight line while moving ball around body (ball size should be adapted to the child's age).

   Emphases for observation:

   a. Arm–leg movement coordination
   b. Ability to cross midline
   c. Movement flow (does transferring ball make the child stop).

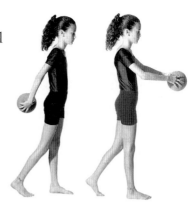

5. Dribbling a basketball

   Instructions: Standing in place, bouncing a basketball sequentially (dribbling).

   Emphases for observation:

   a. Movement flow
   b. Eye–hand coordination
   c. Correct timing in pushing the ball down
   d. Regulation of force.

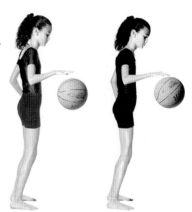

6. Raising opposing arms–legs lying face down

   Instructions: Lying face down both arms forward. Raising one leg and opposite arm at the diagnostician's command.

   Emphases for observation:

   a. Coordination of arm–leg movements
   b. Test of muscle tone in the limbs remaining on the ground (heightened tone may indicate difficulty in regulating force and isolating movement).

7. Crawling in a straight line

   Instructions: Crawling straight forward under an elastic band hanging 30–40 cm from the ground.

   Emphases for observation:

   a. Coordination of arm–leg movements
   b. Movement flow.

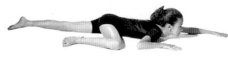

Figure 7.17 *(continued)*.

Balance

The ability to maintain equilibrium and stabilize the body in various starting positions is a precondition for normal balance in both static and dynamic states. As people are usually in movement, they must respond to each movement task with an appropriate dynamic process. To maintain stability while stationary, the body's center of gravity should remain above its base of support. Every movement changes the position of the center of gravity, and postural muscles work to stabilize and organize the body in self spatial orientation and in general spatial orientation.

Difficulties in balance may occur as a result of functional disorders in one or more of the systems in charge (Fig. 7.18). Impairment to the optimal function of each of these systems affects the balance ability in various ways according to the following possibilities:

- Balance difficulties arising from impaired nervous system functioning (problem in obtaining information from the environment, processing the information received or planning correct movement patterns through neural paths to body limbs)
- Balance difficulties resulting from imbalance between antagonistic muscle groups throughout the body
- Balance difficulties because of poor joint positioning (mainly in the lower extremities) and postural disorders.

Distributing body weight evenly over the entire base of support on the foot is extremely important. To this end, there is a need to check for excessive tension or pressure on one part of the foot in comparison to other areas. Such a condition may cause imbalance in higher areas of the body as well as indirectly impairing balance ability.

The messages carried by the peripheral nerves receive information from the sensory organs and send commands to the skeletal muscles, but for fine and precise movement control, the muscles provide constant feedback of information and continual adjustment of motor responses even after they begin their operation. Thus, there exists interrelationship between the nervous system and the musculoskeletal system in various functions requiring balance. Diagnosticians should be aware of the effects of these systems and try to identify the source of the problem.

In psychomotor diagnosis, therapists have the opportunity to diagnose functional imbalance according to how children respond physically to

---

Systems that help maintain balance

Skeletal system
Normal position of joints (optimal load on base of support)

Nervous system
Reception of information ⟶ Information processing ⟶ Determining movement patterns

- Visual information
- Kinesthetic information
- Information from vestibular mechanism in internal ear

Muscular system
Functional balance between antagonistic muscles

Figure 7.18 The systems that help maintain balance (Solberg, 1998a).

forces acting on them. Correct and balanced responses require the ability to use body forces effectively while maintaining balance.

As balance ability is reflected in both static and dynamic situations, diagnosticians should examine both static balance (in diverse starting positions) and dynamic balance. The tests presented here are examples of examination options, and can certainly be altered at the diagnostician's discretion. Special attention has been paid to simple tests that are easy to implement and that provide information in as little time as possible with no need for special apparatus.

The tests examine static and dynamic balance, either separately or together. The children are barefoot as they perform the various tasks so that diagnosticians can obtain important additional information about foot function and ankle joint position, and identify various postural disorders in the feet (see Ch. 5).

However, diagnosticians must also remember that performing tasks barefoot raises the difficulty level because of the smaller base of support.

Tests to evaluate balance

1. Walking a straight line
   Instructions: Walking on a straight line marked on the floor, forwards, backwards and sideways.
   Emphases for observation:

   a. Number of deviations from the line
   b. Directions of deviations from the line
   c. Foot position (toe-in/toe-out, foot arches, etc.).

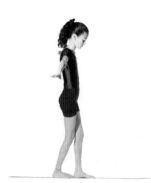

2. Moving forward and stopping on the line
   Instructions: Advancing along a straight line or balance beam 10 cm wide at a height of 10–30 cm (depending on child's age). Occasionally the child is told to stop for a few seconds.
   Emphases for observation:

   a. Dynamic and static balance ability on the beam
   b. Is the movement characterized by shaking, extra movements and excessive trunk swaying from side to side?
   c. Self-confidence in movement.

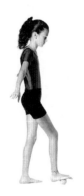

Figure 7.19 Tests to evaluate balance.

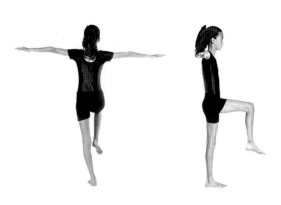

3. Standing on one leg (static balance)
   Instructions: Balancing the body while standing on one foot, arms extended at shoulder level.
   Emphases for observation:

   a. Static balance on one foot

   b. Check of ankle joint stability and the "response" of the support foot. Amount of muscular energy invested in the support foot (is it characterized by much movement near the toes?)

   c. Checking balance in other body parts. Do the pelvic area and trunk manifest excessive movements and swaying to maintain balance? Is the body balanced and still or in constant movement?

In cases where children have difficulty performing this test, it is recommended to allow them to touch the diagnostician's hand lightly. If this light touch helps the children to become stable, the source of the problem may be kinesthetic difficulties in organizing the body, and not necessarily in mechanisms connected to the postural characteristics mentioned.

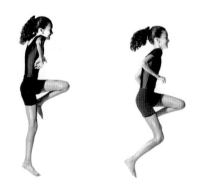

4. Hopping on one foot
   Instructions: Moving forward by hops on one foot.
   Emphases for observation:

   a. Balance ability on one foot during forward movement

   b. Assessment of muscle strength in the hopping foot. Ability to leave the ground and to absorb shocks in the knee and ankle joints when landing.

5. Jumping down into a hoop
   Instructions: Jumping from a height of 50–100 cm (depending on child's age) and landing in a hoop placed on a mattress.
   Emphases for observation:

   a. Checking body's ability to absorb shocks when landing. Does the child succeed in remaining within the hoop area without losing balance?

   b. Checking knee strength in eccentric contraction of the knee extensor muscles

   c. Self-confidence in jumping.

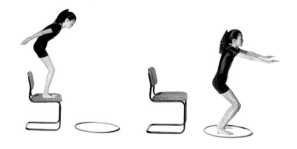

Figure 7.19 (*continued*).

6. Sudden stop

   Instructions: From a fast run – stopping suddenly at a pre-agreed signal.

   Emphases for observation:

   a. Can the child stop immediately and maintain body balance, or does he fall in the effort?

   b. Assessment of reaction time.

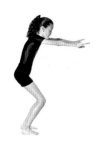

7. Hand–knee stand (six-point stance)

   Instructions:

   - Raising one limb (arm/leg) and stabilizing the body on the other points of support
   - Raising opposing arm and leg
   - Raising arm and leg on same side

   Emphases for observation:

   a. Ability to balance body on various support points for a few seconds

   b. Assessing overall strength in the back and gluteal muscles

   c. Checking ability to balance pelvis and lower back using abdominal muscles

   d. Coordinative ability in differentiating movements.

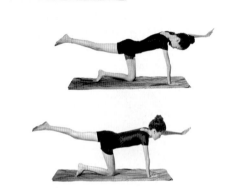

8. Standing on all fours

   Instructions:

   - Raising one limb (arm/leg) and stabilizing body on the remaining points of support
   - Raising opposing arm and leg.

   Emphases for observation:

   a. Ability to balance body on various support points for a few seconds

   b. Assessment of overall strength of shoulder girdle

   c. Coordinative ability in separating movements.

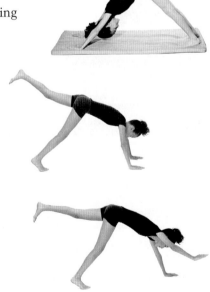

Figure 7.19 *(continued)*.

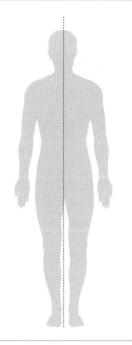

Figure 7.20 Midline of the body.

Crossing the midline

The midline of the body is an imaginary longitudinal line through the center of the body from top to bottom (Fig. 7.20). This line cuts the body into two halves: right side and left side. Crossing the midline refers to the ability to move one part of the body across this line and function in front of the other side of the body.

The ability to cross the midline is based on overall movement control of all the movement components, among them extension, flexion, side flexion and rotation on the horizontal plane (Ratzon, 1993). In normal conditions, children can rotate their trunk easily to both sides, and the arms accompany the movement and work on the facing side. Coordinative problems characterized by the inability to cross the midline may impact negatively on children's general motor functioning. This faulty functioning will appear as motor clumsiness, rigid movement and postural patterns and difficulties in activities of daily living (ADL) such as writing and dressing oneself.

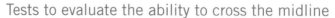

Tests to evaluate the ability to cross the midline

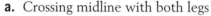

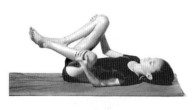

1. Cross walk on a straight line
   Instructions: Walking along a marked straight line, right leg crossing over to left side, and left leg crossing over to right side. Feet should be parallel and next to the marked line.
   Emphases for observation:

   a. Crossing midline with both legs
   b. Balance and width of base of support (distance of feet from the marked line).

2. Rolling from side to side
   Instructions: Lying supine on the back with arms at the sides of the body, rolling from side to side, leading with a different arm each time.
   Emphases for observation:

   a. Crossing midline with arms and legs
   b. Movement flow. Does the movement flow or is it choppy?

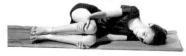

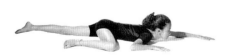

3. Crawling between cones
   Instructions: Crawling between cones set up along a straight line at a distance of 40–60 cm from each other.
   Emphases for observation:

   a. Crossing midline while crawling
   b. Overall movement coordination.

Figure 7.21 Tests to evaluate the ability to cross the midline.

4. Walking in place, hand meeting opposite leg
   Instructions: Stepping in place, raising knees high and bringing each hand in contact with the opposite knee sequentially throughout the movement.
   Emphases for observation:

   a. Ability to cross midline with arm movements
   b. Overall coordination in diagonal movements.

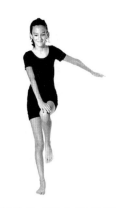

Figure 7.21 *(continued)*.

Basic ball skills

Evaluating children's basic ball skills is part of an integrative approach to functioning and makes it possible to obtain important information about overall motor functioning. Movement with a ball is not an isolated, localized phenomenon. Rather, it occurs in constant coordination with all the other parts of the body. For this reason, working with balls is also an effective and enjoyable means of treatment for improving coordination, force regulation, differentiation of movement, movement timing and accuracy.

Evaluating children's abilities in basic ball skills:

- Catching a ball
- Throwing a ball
- Bouncing a ball (dribbling)
- Shooting a ball to a basket or hoop or pail (depending on child's age).

Emphases for observation:

a. Coordination (arm–leg, eye–hand, eye–foot)
b. Regulation of force, accuracy
c. Differentiation of movement
d. Movement flow and timing
e. Kinesthetic ability.

Gross motor skills

Basic skills are movements children learn to perform as they develop, and on which they will base their future control of their body and their movements. These skills, which include walking, running, jumping, climbing, crawling, rolling, etc., develop naturally in all healthy children, but can be improved by directed experiences and rich motor exposure.

Examination of gross motor skills refers to evaluating children's abilities and functioning in large, general actions. It is recommended that the following skills in this domain be tested in order to obtain information about overall physical functioning.

Tests to evaluate gross motor abilities

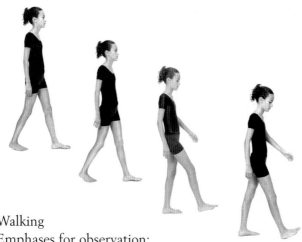

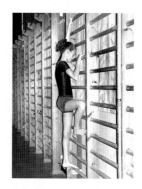

1. Walking
   Emphases for observation:

   a. Movement flow and speed of movement
   b. Base of support (are feet close or far from one another?)
   c. Coordination (do arms and legs swing in opposition or parallel?)
   d. Functioning of feet and ankle joints.

   (Additional parameters for comprehensive diagnosis of the walking cycle are described in Ch. 5).

2. Running
   Emphases for observation:

   a. Coordination
   b. Movement flow (checking for rigidity in muscles of hands, arms, shoulder girdle and face)
   c. Movement speed.

3. Ladder climbing
   Emphases for observation:

   a. Movement planning
   b. Self confidence
   c. Hand grip ability.

4. Forward crawling
   Emphases for observation:

   a. Crossing midline
   b. Coordination
   c. Range of motion in hip joints.

Figure 7.22 Tests to evaluate gross motor abilities.

5. Forward broad jumping
(on two legs)
Emphases for observation:

   a. General strength of lower
   extremities
   b. Balance and ability to stop
   and absorb shocks
   c. Movement coordination
   and timing.

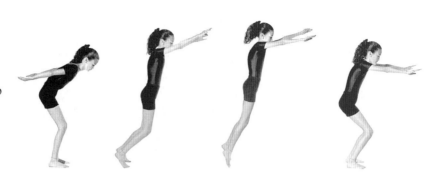

Figure 7.21 (*continued*).

Fine motor skills

Children's fine motor skills are assessed by examining their fine movement functioning, which entails control of small muscle groups. Control of the fine skills requires a high level of movement differentiation, force regulation and movement precision, and is directly connected to the ability to control the trunk and shoulder girdle. Therefore, in cases of fine motor skill difficulties, it is recommended to test the trunk and shoulder girdle because stability in their functioning facilitates control of hand movements (the proximo-distal principle of motor development, see Ch. 12). At times, the source of the difficulty will be identifiable through the hand–trunk–shoulder girdle connection, and treatment can be directed accordingly.

Fine hand movement control is reflected in the ability to produce wrist and finger movements independent of the whole hand. This ability to isolate movement is essential for performing an array of fine skills, such as writing and cutting.

The following are some of the skills that enable therapists to assess children's fine motor functioning. Some of the skills focus on fine motor functions in one hand (drawing, writing), and others test movement coordination between the two hands (beading, tying shoelaces). Some or all of them can be tested, at the diagnostician's discretion.

- Buttoning
- Lacing and unlacing
- Opening and closing zippers
- Stringing beads
- Copying a coin on paper
- Drawing or writing (depending on the child's age).

Emphases for observation in performing the various skills:

- Eye–hand coordination and eye focus
- Ability to differentiate movement, force regulation and accuracy
- Overall strength in hand functioning
- Child's range of attention and concentration.

Other areas of reference in psychomotor diagnosis

Agility and movement speed

Children's overall functioning in daily activities is affected, among other things, by their ability to execute tasks requiring agility and movement speed; therefore, these aspects of movement should be tested as part of the process of motor skill assessment. Children's movement agility is measured, among other things, by their ability to change physical position while changing direction during a rapid movement, both in self-spatial orientation (for example, the rapid transition from lying to standing), and in general spatial orientation (for instance, the ability to change direction rapidly, effectively, and purposefully while running).

Difficulty in these movement aspects may be reflected in situations in which children's motor responses are not appropriate to the demands of the situation they are in. Their movements will be characterized by heaviness, they tend to avoid physical activities requiring rapid and agile movement (such as ball games), and at times this situation may cause lack of self confidence and low self esteem.

Spatial orientation

Spatial orientation is a first step towards developing motor ability. Spatial perception is a process of recognizing different movement terms, location, amplitude, and directionality. It is based on a familiarity with one's body, how the body moves about in its own immediate surroundings and how it moves about in relation to others in the surroundings (Ratzon, 1993), e.g., above–below, up–down, left side-middle–right side, large–small, etc.

Spatial orientation can be divided into two main components:

1. *Self spatial orientation*: This refers to the child's understanding of the movement options available for his body limbs on the various movement planes, while internalizing functional relationships between those body limbs. For example, he will understand that he can bring his chin to his knee, but that he can't "kiss" his back.

   Self-spatial orientation is learned through children's experiences and activities with their bodies, and when necessary, it can be improved through exercises such as identifying and bringing different limbs together, learning the movement options for a given joint in relation to others, etc.

2. *General spatial orientation*: This refers to the individual's place in his environment: moving away–moving towards, going up–going down, entering–exiting, etc. The surroundings are perceived basically through the experience and activity in them, when infants begin to crawl, to "go into", "climb onto", "reach", etc. (Ratzon, 1993).

Disorders in these aspects of self and general spatial orientation may be characterized by clumsy movements. There is a tendency to drop things and to bang into people and objects. Such children tend to fall, and often experience difficulties in daily functions such as dressing themselves, washing up, etc.

Kinesthesis – the feeling of movement

Normal movement patterns in daily actions are based on individuals' ability to feel their body limbs and to control various movement components without the need for visual feedback.

Kinesthesia as a perceptual system allows one to maintain normal posture in static situations and in movement when one is aware of the location of the body limbs and is able to regulate the muscle force applied during activation of these limbs.

The main traits of kinesthetic ability were explained earlier, where details were given of the receptors that facilitate the feeling of movement (Golgi, Rafini, and Pacini receptors, see Ch. 2). These receptors help to maintain posture and absorb information about movement location, range of motion and rhythm. This important functional aspect is reflected in almost every motor action, whether in sports or in daily functioning.

Kinesthetic ability develops over the years and is based on previous motor experiences. Disabilities in this domain lead to the development of postural disorders, low movement quality and motor clumsiness.

Body image

Body image is related to the many aspects of how people see their body and how they internalize functional ties between various body limbs.

Body image is shaped gradually over the years, and it is the product of a large array of factors such as control of body movements and knowing the names and positions of the body limbs. Rich motor exposure and varied movement experience contribute to this process of shaping body image and raising individuals' awareness of their body.

Self esteem

The psychomotor diagnosis and the physical and verbal interactions with the child during diagnosis enable diagnosticians to obtain a picture of a given child's self esteem as well. Self esteem is nourished by body image but many other factors are also involved in shaping it.

In this respect, diagnosticians should test whether a child's self esteem is realistic in terms of real skills: does the child exaggerate in estimating personal ability or tend to underestimate true worth, not believing that he or she can succeed in performing any task even though the capability exists?

The behavioral–emotional aspect The holistic approach in diagnosis makes it possible to obtain important information even about aspects not directly related to a child's physical functioning. Diagnosis and activity create conditions for getting to know the child and for testing his responses to success and to failure. The various stimuli to which the child is exposed during the diagnosis allow him to express his successes, difficulties and frustrations, which usually consist of a broad array of feelings and emotions (Holon Center for Therapeutic Sport, 2000).

Recommended reference points

- Communication – does the child develop ties easily? Is he reachable or otherwise, does he feel comfortable or afraid, does he have trouble being separated from his parents, etc.?
- Self confidence – does the child need constant confirmation and reinforcement for his actions? Does he express fear while performing tasks that require little courage? Does he speak confidently and express himself freely? Does he make eye contact with the diagnostician, etc.?
- Frustration threshold – how does the child respond to difficulty? Does he tend to give up or does he make more effort and insist on succeeding?
- Expressing feeling – does the child cry or laugh a lot? Does he exhibit nervousness or general joyfulness? Does he experience extreme mood swings? Does he demand contact with the diagnostician, or reject him?
- Cooperation and motivation – is the child apathetic and unmotivated, or does he cooperate and reveal motivation and enthusiasm even in less interesting tasks?
- Cognition – does the child understand movement terms, movement directions, shapes, colors, etc.? Does he have difficulty understanding complex tasks and performing them? Does he have a rich language?
- Concentration and attention – is the child restless in his movements? Is he easily distracted? Does he show a tendency to "jump" from place to place? Does he have a short concentration span? Does he wait patiently for the end of the explanation before performing the task?

In terms of the subject of this chapter, these behavioral–emotional aspects are presented as a means for getting to know the child, but at the same time, it should be remembered that the diagnostic emphasis depends on the type of problem and the information received from the parents (see the first stage of the diagnosis). The behavioral–emotional aspects presented here for testing can be further developed, expanded and emphasized as needed.

Summarizing psychomotor diagnosis data

This section presents a table for summarizing data (Table 2). The purpose of Table 2 is to focus on overall assessment in each domain of the diagnosis, without recording a specific evaluation for each test. The assumption is that a correct professional diagnostic view will create "crosschecks of information" obtained from observations of the various tasks in a given area, thus enabling the diagnostician to give an overall evaluation in that domain.

This approach will help map the desired directions the treatment should take and ways to implement them. This simplification should help diagnosticians or therapists to avoid having to deal with overly detailed data.

As noted, the assessment is subjective and on a scale of 1 (the weakest level of functioning) to 5 (the highest level of functioning). Overall evaluation in each domain is based on a battery of tests for the same skill with reference to the various emphases during observation.

To summarize, presentation of the ways of diagnosing postural disorders indicates the recommended approach during the treatment stage as well, in which the child should not be seen as a mass of joints, muscles, and bones. The most important component is the child's personality that connects and is "connected" to those joints. Therefore, it is not enough to perform a posture examination; it is necessary to expose the child to a variety of tasks that will reveal not only the physical sides but also other elements in his or her personality. These elements, pertaining to the child's social, emotional, and cognitive status, may also indicate the source of a given problem and help to select the correct emphases in treatment.

And above all, the general information obtained helps therapists to become acquainted with the child, to come close to him, to create an atmosphere of trust, and of course, to use the material that is revealed about his personality to build an exercise program that will bond to his inner world. This approach, which places the child's personality and not problematic joints in the spotlight, should be emphasized in adapted physical activity and in other disciplines related to paramedical treatment.

Table 7.2 Assessment of psychomotor functioning: summary table of diagnostic data

TEST AREA	1 VERY WEAK	2 WEAK	3 MODERATE	4 GOOD	5 VERY GOOD	QUALITATIVE ASSESSMENT OF MOVEMENT PATTERNS
A. BASIC SKILLS						
Crawling						
Walking						
Running						
Climbing						
Jumping on two feet						
Hopping on right foot						
Hopping on left foot						
Skipping						
Forward somersault						
B. BALL SKILLS						
Passing (throwing)						
Catching						
Bouncing						
Shooting						
Kicking a soccer ball						
Stopping a soccer ball						
Shoulder throw with a small ball						
C. FINE MOTOR SKILLS						
Buttoning						
Tying shoelaces						
Writing						
Control of fingers						
D. GENERAL MOTOR ABILITIES						
Static balance on right leg						
Static balance on left leg						
Dynamic balance						
Agility						
Speed						
General coordination						
Eye/hand coordination						
Timing						
Regulation of force						
Reaction time						
Movement flow						
Crossing midline						
General spatial orientation						
Personal spatial orientation						
Kinesthesis – feeling of movement						

GENERAL ASSESSMENT

Table 7.2 Assessment of psychomotor functioning: summary table of diagnostic data (*continued*)

TEST AREA	1 VERY WEAK	2 WEAK	3 MODERATE	4 GOOD	5 VERY GOOD	QUALITATIVE ASSESSMENT OF MOVEMENT PATTERNS
E. BEHAVIORAL–EMOTIONAL–COGNITIVE CHARACTERISTICS						
Concentration and attention						
Cooperation and motivation						
General cognitive ability						
Language and speech						
Self confidence						
Self image						
Body image						
Motor memory						
Movement planning						
Distinguishing right and left						

F. GENERAL EVALUATION

G. MAIN EMPHASES FOR TREATMENT

1.

2.

3.

4.

CHAPTER 8

Therapeutic exercise — specific areas of practice

Doing therapeutic exercises to improve posture should follow the shower principle: better 10 minutes each day than 1 hour once a week

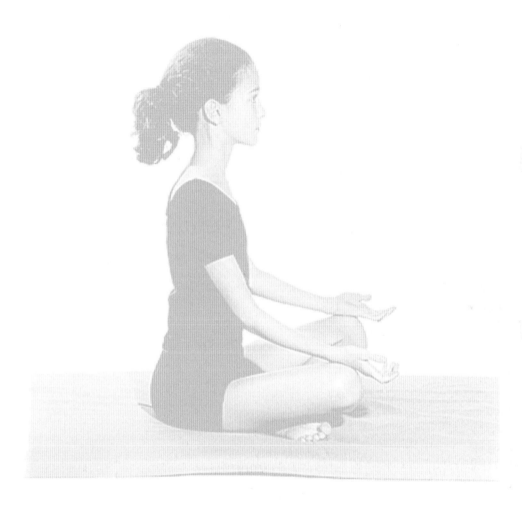

One of the basic principles of working correctly and safely is to plan balanced activity that helps to maintain both muscle strength and flexibility. Aside from the genetic code that determines postural patterns, muscle length and strength are very important factors in overall functioning. While heritage traits affect mainly the osseous structure of the skeleton, and especially of the spinal column, the muscles determine the position of the joints in relation to the line of gravity.

As mentioned previously, joint position is a function of the relative strength of antagonist muscles. Imbalance between groups of antagonist muscles alters the balance of forces exerted on the specific joints and affects their position. An integral part of therapeutic exercise involves bringing muscles to the appropriate length and strength for maintaining optimal posture and function. This chapter will present examples of exercises for the areas most relevant to the locomotor system and posture.

Exercises to lengthen the hamstring muscles

The thigh extensor group located behind the thigh and collectively known as the hamstrings includes three muscles:

- Biceps femoris
- Semitendinosus
- Semimembranosus

The origins and insertions of these muscles are detailed in Chapter 2.

The hamstrings pass over two joints, and their tendency to shorten is connected both to their involvement in various functions such as walking, running, climbing steps, etc., and to how they function. For example, in static situations such as sitting, one end remains in a shortened state for long periods of time (Gur, 1999a).

A shortening of these muscles will restrict thigh flexion or knee extension, but the adverse functional effects will also include the pelvis and the lumbar spine (Fig. 8.1). Thus, hamstring stretching exercises are also intended, indirectly, to improve mobility of the pelvis and the lower back (Gould & Davies, 1985).

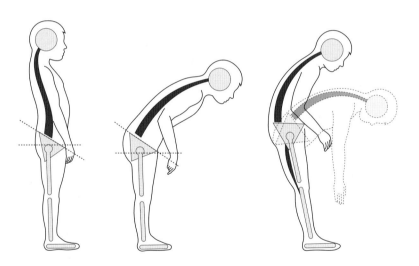

Figure 8.1 Effect of hamstrings on the pelvis and lower back in forward flexion (lumbo-pelvic rhythm). As the range of flexion increases, so too does involvement of the hip joints, and the stretching ability of the hamstrings is more essential (Gur, 1999b). In daily functioning, their normal flexibility helps to reduce loads exerted on the lower back.

Exercises 1 and 2 focus on initial stretching of the muscles (over only one joint) as a basis for stretching them throughout the range of motion in exercises 3–10.

1. Lying on back – holding one knee with both hands and nearing it to chest.

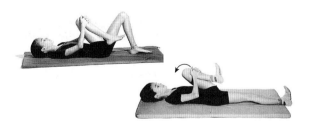

2. Lying on back – using the hands to bring both knees towards the chest.

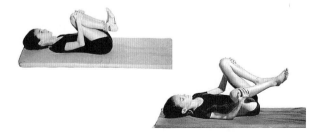

Figure 8.2 Exercises to lengthen the hamstring muscles.

3. Lying on back – feet close to pelvis. Bringing one knee to the chest and straightening the leg upward with dorsiflexion of foot.

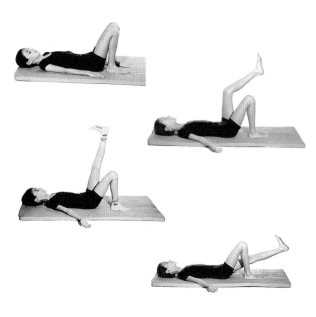

4. Lying on back – knees to abdomen and support cushion under pelvis. Straightening both legs and stretching them upwards.

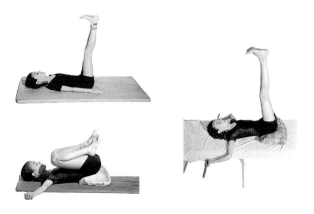

5. Sitting up with legs straight out – hands providing ground support behind the back. Pushing the floor while tilting the torso forward and performing anterior pelvic tilt (APT) until there is a feeling of stretch in the hamstrings.

6. Sitting – one leg straight and the other flexed, bringing heel to groin. One hand on the floor behind and the second moves along the straight leg with a slight forward bending of the torso.

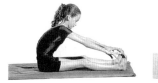 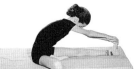

7. Standing on hands and knees – bringing one foot between hands, and from here, rocking the body forward and backward releasing head and leaning chest on thigh.

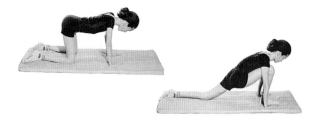

8. Four point stand – head between arms and heels in the air. Tilting body weight towards the hands, and then straightening knees and lowering both heels towards the floor.

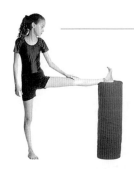

9. Standing in front of a table, chair (or other support) – raising one leg and statically stretching the hamstrings.

10. Lying on side, bringing knees to chest – arms straight out in front of face. Straightening upper leg to the side.

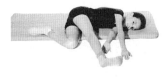

Figure 8.2 (continued).

Exercises to lengthen lower back muscles

The build-up of stress in the lower back may cause discomfort and pain. The smaller than normal range of motion in this area creates a functioning limitation and with time the lack of movement may result in degenerative changes in the lumbar vertebrae. The following exercises are intended to fulfill the need to maintain the lower back mobility and prevent excessive muscle tone in this area.

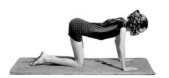 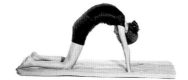 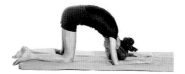

1. **a.** Standing on hands and knees – while exhaling, contracting the abdomen and concaving the back while bringing chin to chest.

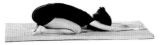 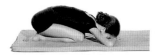

b. Lowering pelvis to heels and forehead to the floor.

c. Fetal position – pelvis to heels, forehead to floor, and hands under forehead (static position for lower back relaxation).

2. Crossed legs sitting – moving hands forward while bending the torso and lowering the forehead towards the floor.

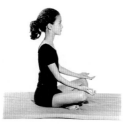 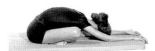

3. Crossed legs sitting – moving one hand forward while flexing the torso in different directions.

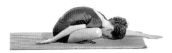 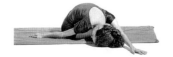 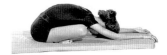

Figure 8.3 Exercises to lengthen lower back muscles.

4. Lying on back – feet on floor near pelvis. Posterior pelvic tilt (PPT) while holding in the abdomen during exhalation and flattening the lower back.

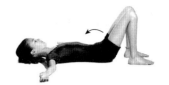

5. **a.** Lying on back – feet on floor. Using hands to bring one knee towards chest and slowly draw it towards the body. After a few attempts, it is possible to straighten the second leg.

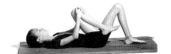 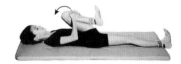

   b. Using hands to bring both knees towards the chest.

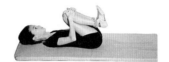 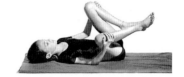

   c. Hands provide support on the ground. Gradually bringing knees towards forehead and lowering the back slowly towards the floor – without using hands.

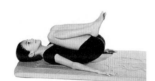 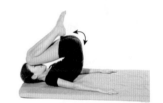

   d. Holding knees in hands – rolling the body from side to side.

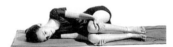 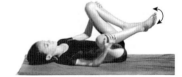

   e. "Seesaw" – rolling forward and backward.

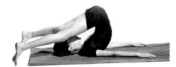 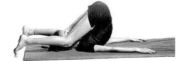 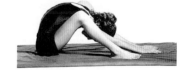

6. Lying on back – hands extended to the sides at shoulder height, and knees bent to abdomen. Lowering the knees slowly from side to side.

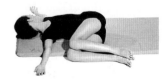

Figure 8.3 (*continued*).

Spine lengthening exercises (traction)

Spinal traction is included in this chapter on postural exercises because of its positive effect on the musculoskeletal system while treating various postural disorders (Heijden et al., 1995).

Various therapy methods employ manipulations and special apparatus to stretch joints. At the same time, it is possible to create a spinal traction effect by means of exercises that utilize appropriate starting points.

Spinal traction exercises can be used for a number of purposes:

1. To stretch spinal muscles and ligaments.
2. To expand intervertebral gaps and to separate vertebrae from one other.
3. To reduce spinal curves.
4. To reduce pressure exerted on intervertebral discs (in cases of pathologies in the intervertebral discs).

Spinal traction in operation

Several methods can be employed for stretching the spinal vertebrae lengthwise. In terms of movement, there are two main approaches:

1. Holding a static position for prolonged periods, depending on the patient's sensations (Kisner & Colby, 1985).
2. Integrating movement in traction activity.

The examples given in this chapter emphasize the use of traction as an integral part of postural exercises, and because ultimately patients should perform these exercises independently, it is important to adopt methods that are suited to their needs and abilities.

The examples in this chapter employ traction in static conditions so as to create a stretching effect and general lengthening of the entire spinal column without focusing on specific vertebral areas. It should be emphasized that in all of the exercises, the pelvis should be tilted posteriorly.

- In treating acute conditions (back pains, ruptured discs and/or disorders involving nervous damage), traction exercises should be employed under medical supervision only.

Figure 8.4 presents examples of starting positions that facilitate overall stretching (traction) of the spinal column.

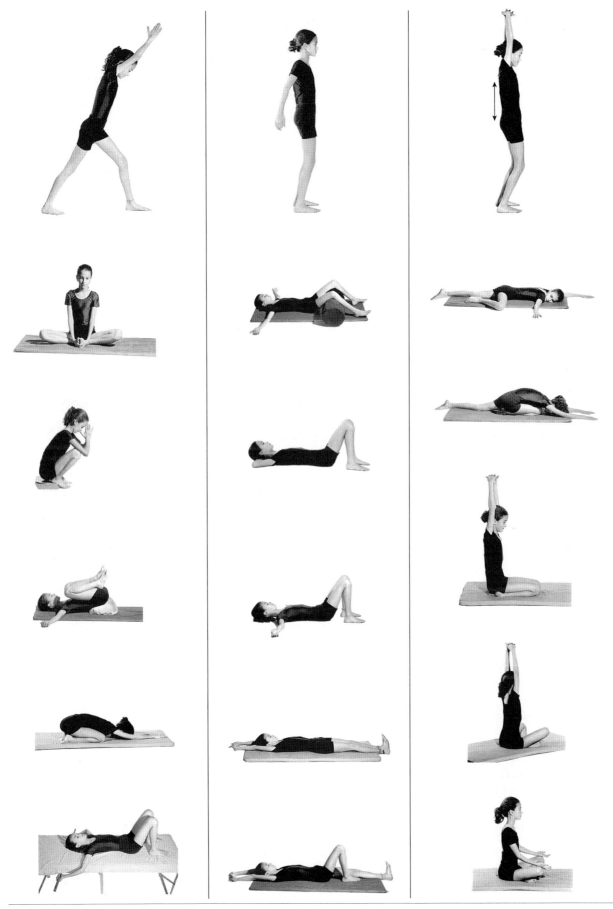

Figure 8.4 Spine lengthening exercises (traction).

Exercises to lengthen chest muscles

Chest muscles are one of the main facilitators of a good range of shoulder girdle motion. A shortening of the chest muscles will limit the options for moving the shoulder (mainly arm extension) and in some cases will create a tendency towards postural disorders (kyphosis).

Lengthening these muscles (pectoralis major/pectoralis minor) will reduce the resistance of the back muscles (antagonists) and will allow the scapulae to remain in their correct position without being pulled forward.

1. Lying on back with knees bent – stretching arms from the sides backwards and lowering them from a raised position. Performing variations of the movement (cushion under knees, knees bent to chest, legs straight on the ground).

2. **a.** Lying on back – arms stretched to sides at shoulder height and knees bent to abdomen. Lowering knees slowly from side to side.
   b. Lowering knees to the side and holding them static (emphasis on deep breathing while holding the position).

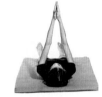

   c. Hands under head for support, elbows on floor. Lowering knees from side to side.

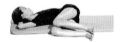
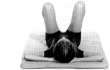

   d. Moving elbow from side to side (opening and closing movements of the thorax).

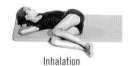
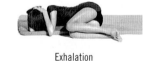

Inhalation   Exhalation

3. Lying on side, knees bent to chest; arms straight out to the side, at face level – creating circular movements (with upper arm) around the body with head moving in same direction.

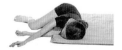
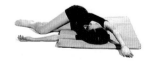

4. **a.** Lying on narrow bench (or other raised surface) – arms raised (hand to hand), then lowering them straight to sides and holding passively.
   b. Making circles with both arms.
   c. After a few times, stretching with hands under head while lowering elbows.

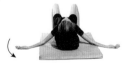
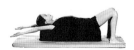
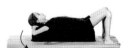

Figure 8.5 Exercises to lengthen chest muscles.

5. Lying on bench, knees bent, hands holding a stick under the bench – straightening and stretching arms, and flexing them until scapulae are brought towards each other.

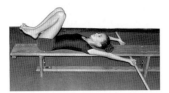 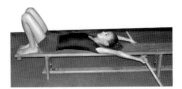 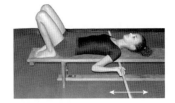

6. **a.** Lying face down, forehead or cheek on floor, fingers clasped above pelvis – raising clasped hands upwards. Cushion under abdomen.

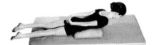 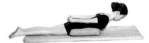

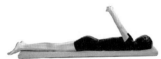

   b. Raising back while pulling hands back and adducting scapulae.

7. Standing on hands and knees, with hands laid on raised bench (or cushion) and head relaxed – lowering pelvis towards heels until there's a feeling of stretch in the chest area.

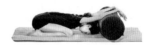 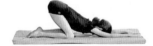

8. Crossed legs sitting – arms straight together in front of body at face level – during inhalation extending arms to sides and adducting scapulae. Performing other variations as in the pictured movements.

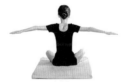

9. Standing – stretching one arm upward and the second backwards (stretching obliques).

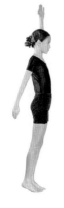

10. Standing – one arm straight forward at face level. Extending arm to side and backwards (at shoulder level), while rotating torso in the direction of the movement.

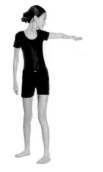 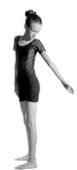

Figure 8.5 (*continued*).

Exercises to strengthen back muscles

Some postural disorders are the result of weak back muscles. The erector spinae keep the spine erect and prevent it from falling forward. The scapulae adductors should be strong enough to prevent the scapulae from being drawn forward, a condition that may cause round and slumped shoulders.

When performing physical exercises for the back and spinal areas, a few important factors should be kept in mind:

- Spinal stability depends on muscular activity. The erector spinae, which protect spinal erectness against the pull of gravity, require high levels of endurance. Their mode of operation in daily functioning requires them to perform over extended periods of time and against relatively low resistance. Therefore, it is recommended to find ways to activate them in a manner that matches what is expected of them, that is, to have them work against low resistance for long periods and with many repetitions

- The erector spinae in the lumbar area have a tendency to "shorten", a condition which may cause movement rigidity in the lower back and pains later on. This should be kept in mind when exercising to strengthen the back, and starting positions should be found that hold these muscles in their lengthened state (that is, in starting positions that emphasize posterior pelvic tilt) (Fig. 8.7)

- To strengthen the back muscles properly and integratively, they should be activated at many execution angles. Therefore, it is advisable to perform many variations of many different exercises that activate the back muscles in various modes

- To prevent excessive loads on the lower back, care should be taken with exercises that work with large 'levers' where the axis of movement is in the pelvic area (Fig. 8.6).

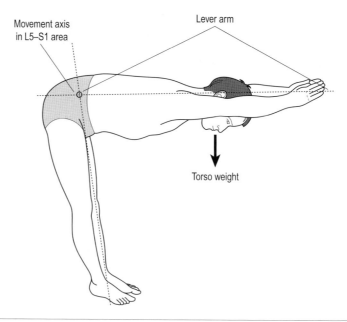

Figure 8.6 Creating large loads on the lower back by using a large lever in moving the body forward.

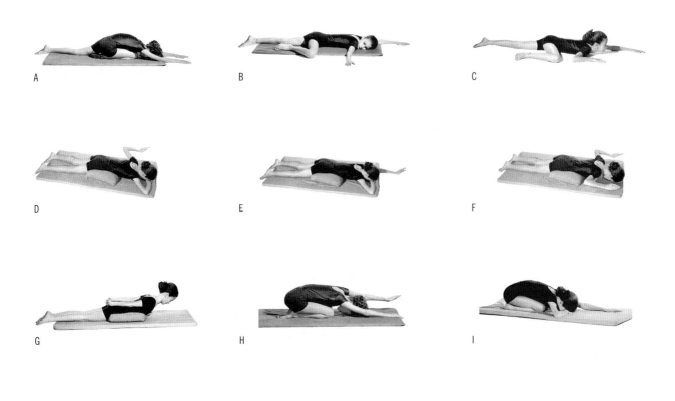

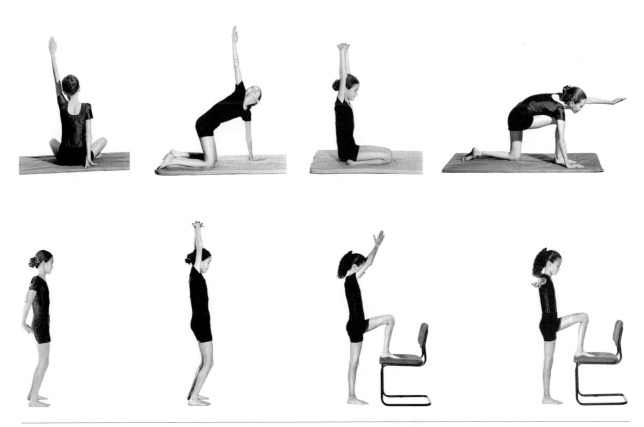

Figure 8.7 Examples of starting positions that help strengthen lower back muscles in their lengthened position.

Most of the exercises lying face down should be performed with a support cushion under the abdomen.

1. **a.** Lying face down, cushion under abdomen, one hand under forehead, the second straight forward – raising arm straight up (without lifting head) and lowering to floor.

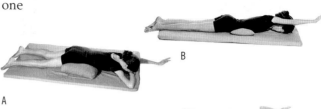

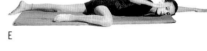

b. After raising arm – flexing elbow towards the torso while contracting the scapulae adductors on the same side.

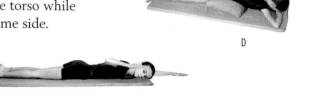

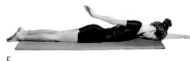

c. The same movements as above with one knee flexed to the side (same side).

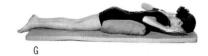

d. Raising straight arm up, moving it in the air along the body and returning to the front (as in freestyle swimming motion).

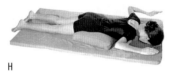

e. Flexing elbows and adducting scapulae on both sides with forehead on ground.

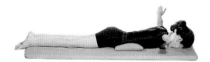

2. **a.** Lying face down, cushion under abdomen, forehead on floor and arms stretched out to sides – raising arms while adducting scapulae towards each other, without raising forehead from floor.

b. Raising arms along body and lifting forehead from floor while pressing chin to chest.

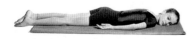
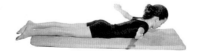
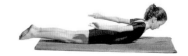

Figure 8.8 Exercises to strengthen back muscles.

3. **a.** Crossed legs sitting, one arm supporting body on floor from behind – raising other arm while lengthening the torso and lowering the arm to the side.

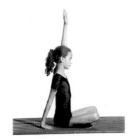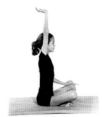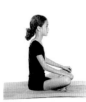

b. Raising both arms while lengthening the torso and pulling in the abdomen. While lowering hands to the sides, relaxing the upper torso and creating a slight forward arching.

c. Sitting with feet facing each other. While inhaling: lengthening the torso. While exhaling: relaxation of the torso with a slight forward arching.

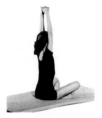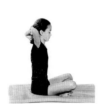

4. **a.** Standing on hands and knees – lowering pelvis to heels, forehead to floor, arms forward. Raising one arm straight ahead and slowly lowering to floor.

b. Hands under forehead. Raising elbows from floor (without breaking hand contact) and contracting scapulae adductors.

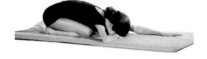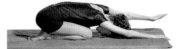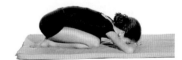

5. **a.** Standing on hands and knees – raising one arm straight forward and lowering slowly to floor.

b. Raising arm and leg on same side. Or opposite sides.

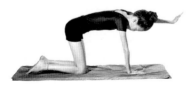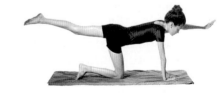

6. Lying on back – hands under pelvis. Contracting both scapulae, bringing them close together, and releasing.

It is recommended to perform with support cushion under head.

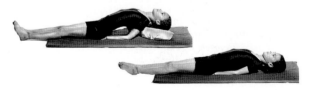

Figure 8.8 (*continued*).

Exercises to strengthen abdominal muscles

Pelvic position and stability directly affect spinal position in general, and especially of the lumbar vertebrae. The main factors that facilitate pelvic stabilization are muscles and ligaments, and the basis for pelvic balance is a balance between antagonist muscle groups responsible for its movement on the sagittal plane (anterior and posterior pelvic tilt) (Solberg, 1996a).

The abdominal muscles play an important role in maintaining pelvic stability. Weakness in these muscles may cause excessive anterior pelvic tilt, which (in a chain effect) adversely affects lower back stability (abdominal weakness – impaired pelvic stability – anterior pelvic tilt – increased lumbar lordosis) (also see Ch. 2, Fig. 2.22).

The recommended exercises emphasize contraction of the abdominal muscles with posterior pelvic tilt.

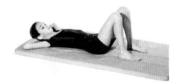

1. Lying on back – hands on back of head and feet on floor.

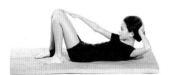

b. During exhalation – raising head until scapulae leave floor. Elbows are parallel to floor without creating an arch in the upper back. During inhalation – returning slowly to the floor.

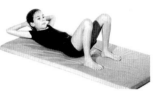

a. During exhalation – bringing one arm towards knees.

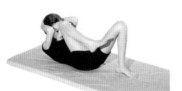

d. During exhalation – raising head while bringing two knees to elbows.

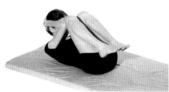

c. During exhalation – bringing one knee to chest and elbows to knee. During inhalation – returning slowly to floor.

e. During exhalation – raising head using hands, bringing knees to forehead and straightening one or both legs upward.

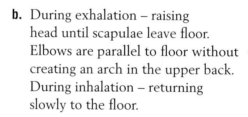

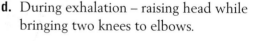

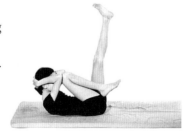

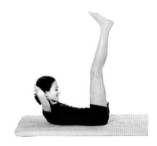

Figure 8.9 Exercises to strengthen abdominal muscles.

2. **a.** Lying on back, arms on sides of body and feet on floor – during exhalation, bringing knees to chest and raising pelvis slightly (the movement can be continued until knees reach forehead and from there are returned slowly and with control to the floor).

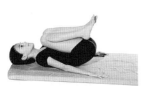
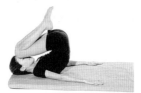

    b. Same as above, with hands supporting the back of the head, and elbows on floor.

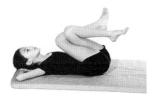
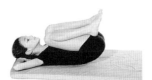

3. Standing on hands and knees – convexing back while contracting abdominal and lower pelvic muscles. To prevent overload on the wrist, this exercise can be performed with forearms on floor.

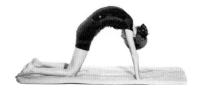
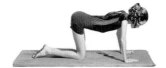
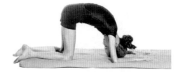

4. Crossed legs sitting – exhaling while gathering in abdomen and contracting lower pelvic muscles.

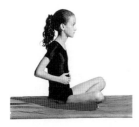
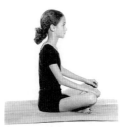

Figure 8.9 (*continued*).

Exercises to improve foot functioning

The foot is the base of body posture. It supports the entire body and makes it possible to maintain balance in both static positions (standing) and in movement (walking, running, ascending, and descending stairs, etc.).

The arched structure of the foot is composed of a longitudinal arch and a transverse arch (see Ch. 2). In addition to providing elasticity, these arches strengthen the feet and make them better at shock absorption. The arches on the feet are maintained thanks to the structure of bones, ligaments and muscles (Norkin & Levangie, 1993).

Improper foot position may cause postural disorders and impact upon motor functions that rely on balance. The aims of the following exercises are to improve foot functioning, prevent weakness by strengthening the intrinsic muscles, and improve blood flow (Solberg, 1996b).

These exercises should be performed barefooted.

1. Sitting

   a. Passively moving the foot in different directions (using hands).
   b. Massaging the foot.

2. Sitting, leaning back on hands

   a. Circular movements of the feet.
   b. Alternate dorsi- and plantar flexion.

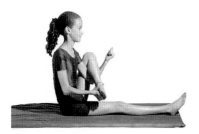

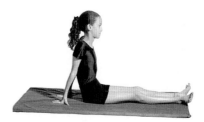

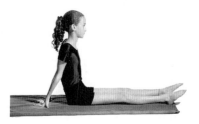

Figure 8.10 Exercises to improve foot functioning.

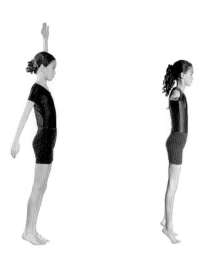

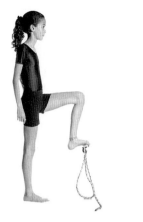

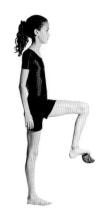

3. **a.** Standing – rising on toes and slowly descending.

b. Grasping small objects with toes (skip rope, bean bag, sock, pieces of paper).

c. Walking on toes.

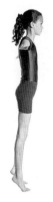

d. Standing – transferring center of gravity backward or forward without breaking heel contact with floor. Knees straight or flexed.

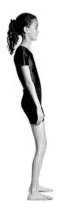

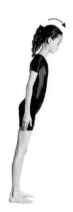

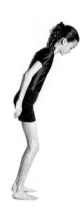

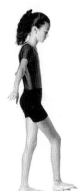

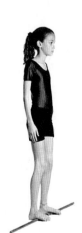

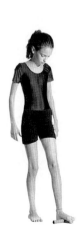

e. Rolling foot on a wooden stick or a small ball.

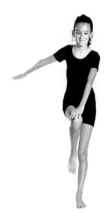

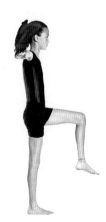

f. Standing on one leg – with variations.

Figure 8.10 *(continued)*.

Exercises to improve balance

The balance mechanism is composed of a group of neuromotor functions and responses that enable individuals to control their movements in various situations (Ratzon, 1993). Balance ability increases slowly and gradually from the initial developmental stages. The process of lifting the pelvis, the torso, and the head above the support base of the legs continues for a long time. Gradually, humans learn to organize their body in balance so that the center of gravity is located above the base of support in both static and dynamic situations.

Balance is the basis for normal posture (see Ch. 7), which is why it must be improved by exercising various movements in different situations. The following exercises are intended to meet this need.

Most of the exercises recommended here should be performed barefooted.

1. Walking a line:

   a. Walking a straight line marked on the ground
   b. Walking a twisting line
   c. Walking a line on the toes (with heels raised)
   d. Walking a straight line, crossing legs.

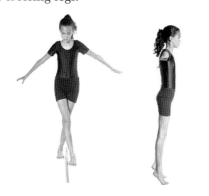

2. Standing on one leg – balancing the body on all the support points of the foot.

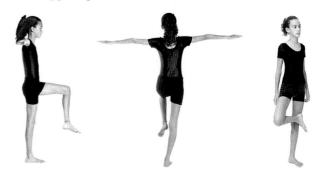

3. Jumps on one leg, while moving forward.

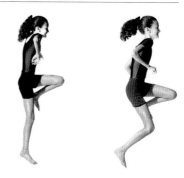

4. Hand–knee stand (six-point stand)

   a. Raising right arm forward and left leg backward
   b. Balancing the body for a few seconds
   c. Returning to hand–knee stand.

   To be performed with both sides of body (opposing arm and leg)
   To be performed with same side arm and leg.

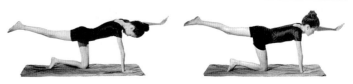

Figure 8.11 Exercises to improve balance.

5. Standing

   a. Stretching one arm up and second arm back (diagonal
      lengthening) while rising on toes

   b. Static hold for a few seconds

   c. Lowering arms along body while lowering heels to floor.

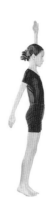

6. Balancing body statically using different bases of support.

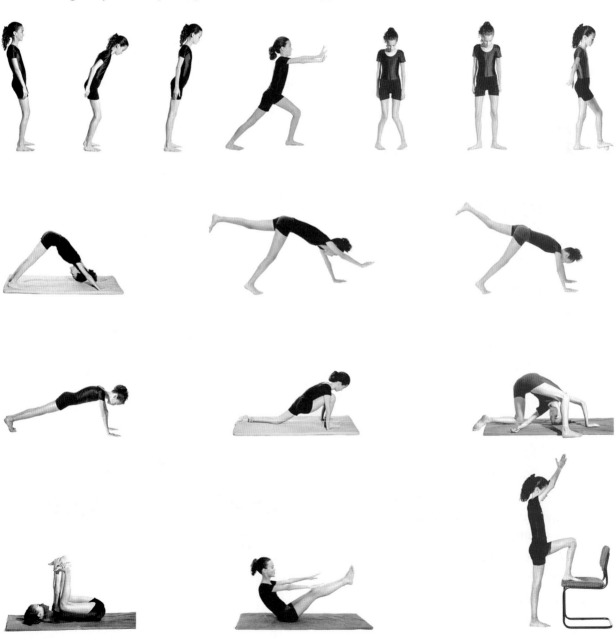

Figure 8.11 (*continued*).

Breathing exercises

Short, shallow breathing impairs overall body functioning and does not utilize the full ability to absorb oxygen. The breathing process entails an expansion of overall chest volume and a diminution of its size by means of the intercostal muscles and the diaphragm. Thus, improper functioning of these muscles as a result of disorders such as kyphosis or scoliosis will also impair optimal functioning of the respiratory system (Solberg, 1996b).

Breathing exercises are also intended to enhance body awareness, which is the basis for any improvement in posture. Some of the following exercises deal with learning and implementing the stages of 'full' breathing in movement.

1. Lying on back, feet on floor and hands on abdomen

   a. Abdominal breathing
   During inhalation – 'inflating' the belly and pushing hands up
   During exhalation – bringing belly back down.

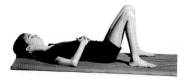

   b. Chest breathing
   Placing hands on the sides of the ribs (as if holding an accordion)
   Inhalation – expanding the chest and ribs and pushing hands to the sides
   Exhalation – pressing hands inward and reducing chest volume.

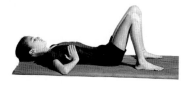

   c. Combining abdominal and chest breathing (full breathing)
   Inhalation – divided into two stages:
   (1) "Inflating" the belly, and (2) expanding chest and ribs
   Exhalation – first drawing in belly, and then reducing chest volume.

   Both inhalation and exhalation should be slow and long.

2. Crossed legged sitting

   a. Abdominal breathing
   b. Chest breathing
   c. Full breathing (according to stages in exercise 1).

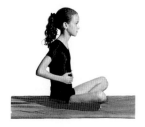

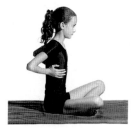

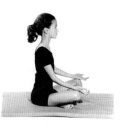

Figure 8.12 Breathing exercises.

3. Crossed legs sitting

 Full inhalation – bringing hands up and interlacing fingers while stretching

 Holding breath for a few seconds while holding in abdomen and lengthening torso upward

 Exhalation – slowly lowering arms to the sides.

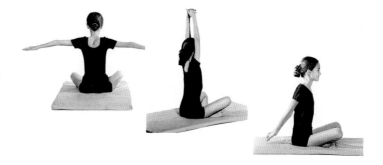

4. Hand–knee stand

 Inhalation – releasing abdomen and arching lower back concavely

 Exhalation – convexing back up and strongly contracting abdomen upward.

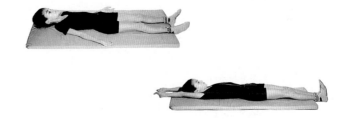

5. Lying on back

 Inhalation – stretching arms to the sides backward

 Holding breath for a few seconds (with lungs full)

 Exhalation – slowly lowering arms.

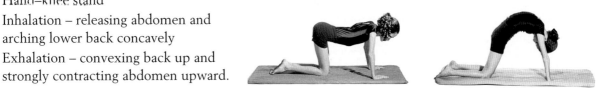

Figure 8.12 (*continued*).

The main emphasis of the exercises presented in this chapter is on body posture and one of the aims is to arrive at a better balance between groups of antagonistic muscles. At the same time, in order to achieve better results (which will not only improve muscle functioning, but also contribute to improved movement and postural patterns in daily functioning), it is not enough to mechanically practice any given exercise. To avoid superficiality, each action should be performed with a conscious awareness of how movement and breathing are coordinated, and an effort should be made to internalize the functional ties between various body limbs and organs.

The practical exercises in this chapter were divided into categories so that teachers or therapists can refer to each specific subject according to their individual needs. In planning a whole movement lesson, and after setting the aim and general direction of it, it is possible to include a variety of exercises from different categories, from an awareness of the particular area that each exercise or position affects more intensively. In any case, it is necessary to prepare the body properly both to avoid damage and to improve results.

As a Chinese sage once said, it is not the sugar that sweetens the tea but the mixing. Here, logical sequencing of the exercises constitutes the most important basis for planning a good, balanced movement lesson.

CHAPTER 9

Special treatment techniques for improving posture and body awareness

Techniques are like noses.
Everybody has one...

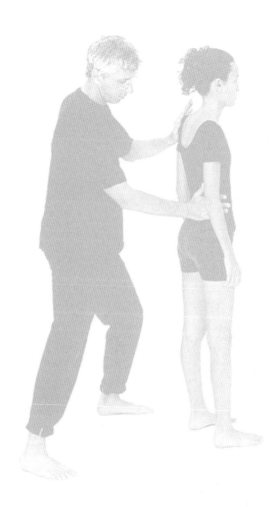

As a result of improper movement patterns over time, one tends to lose the feeling of balance that characterizes normal posture. The focus of attention in such cases is mainly on body awareness. Raising body awareness is the basis for improving overall posture.

"The link system"

In therapeutic exercise, "the link system" is the recommended approach to body movement. This kinesiological principle refers to the mechanism by which the position and function of each joint affects "neighboring" joint function. Thus, a specific movement in a given joint creates a link system that affects the movement or position of another joint.

Using this principle makes it possible to improve the functioning of a given joint and even to relieve pain symptoms by activating "neighboring joints" (indirect treatment). An example of this important kinesiological principle would be lateral rotation of the arm, which indirectly creates retraction (a pulling down and back) of the scapula and thus improves the position of the shoulder girdle in conditions of kyphosis (Fig. 9.1).

Visually, this system looks like a spiral, as illustrated in Figure 9.2.

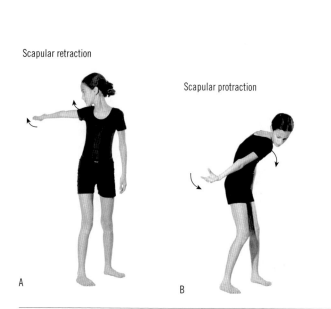

Figure 9.1 Link effect of arm movement on scapular position. (A) Scapular retraction. (B) Scapular protraction.

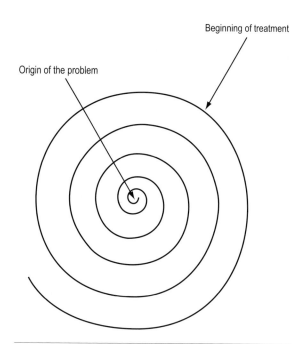

Figure 9.2 The "spiral" as a therapeutic–rehabilitative principle (indirect treatment that makes use of a 'normal' joint to preserve the functioning of a 'faulty' joint).

Using a skip rope to learn and practice pelvic mobility

Proper positioning of the pelvis is a prerequisite for balanced posture alignment on the sagittal plane. Much exercise is required to internalize anterior and posterior pelvic tilt movements and to attain good control when balancing the pelvis in a correct position. Lack of control of this movement usually stems from difficulties in kinesthetic ability, and patients have difficulty placing the pelvis on the basis of movement feelings alone (without visual feedback). Therefore, touch should be made a part of the practice process, to help patients feel their pelvic movement. One means of attaining this touch is a skip rope. As patients lie on their back, with the rope placed beneath their lumbar vertebrae, the exercise goes through the following stages (Fig. 9.3):

Stage 1: Lying – opening arms to the sides and pressing the sacrum to the floor.

Stage 2: The pelvis naturally makes an anterior tilt and creates a space between the back and floor.

Stage 3: The therapist pulls the rope through the lumbar concavity that is created, in a way that the patient feels the rope movement.

Stage 4: Patients are asked to "block" the rope movement and stop it with their back (to do this, patients must find the way to tilt their pelvis posteriorly and neutralize their lumbar lordosis).

In this manner, they can be taught to control their pelvic movement, and after practicing the various stages, they can begin to implement the movement while standing as well.

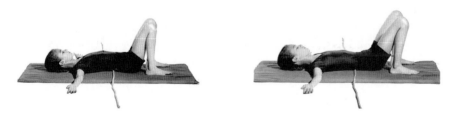

Figure 9.3 Practicing pelvic mobility using a skip rope.

Using a wall to align posture

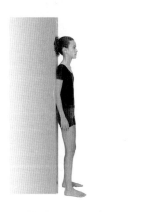

Figure 9.4 Exercising posture with a wall.

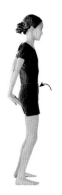

Figure 9.6 Posterior pelvic tilt to reduce lumbar lordosis.

Using a wall may help to improve postural patterns on the sagittal plane and to properly align/organize pelvic, spinal curve, and scapular positions.

The exercises presented here illustrate how to use a wall to balance the body. After performing these exercises, patients may develop a feel for balanced posture and will then be able to perform the movements without a wall to assist them.

After patients learn and perform correct body position, it is recommended to repeat the exercises occasionally using a wall as a means of self examination and of improving pelvic, spinal, thoracic, and scapular positioning.

During the initial stages of practice, patients may experience some difficulty in understanding or carrying out instructions, but experience shows that after the body adjusts to these situations, the exercises can be performed much more easily and naturally with correct and efficient use of the working muscles.

Learning and exercising posture against a wall entails the following stages (Fig. 9.4):

- Standing 10–20 cm from the wall with feet parallel, about pelvic-width distance between them. At this distance, resting the spine on the wall does not give a feeling of "leaning" back (so that if the wall were suddenly removed, no action would be needed to prevent patients from falling backward). Placing the feet in this position allows a balanced distribution of body weight on these points (Fig. 9.5):
  - Five toes
  - Lateral edge of the foot
  - Center of the heel

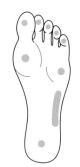

Figure 9.5 Support points on the foot.

- Good balance of body weight on these bases of support strengthens "rooting" the feet in the ground and serves as a basis for improving posture
- The knee joints flex slightly, until the patellae are located exactly above the toes. This position encourages maximal development of strength for exercising
- The pelvis is tilted backward (posterior pelvic tilt – PPT) when the lower back is held close to the wall until there is a feeling that the sacrum is pulling the spine downward (Fig. 9.6)
- Organizing the center of the back – in posterior pelvic tilt, the lower ribs should be pushed towards the wall. This action will cause a feeling of lengthening the central and lower back

- Organizing upper back, neck and head – following PPT, the upper back should be brought as close as possible to the wall without creating tension. The head is held as though pushed back gently, and at the same time the center of the skull is raised (Fig. 9.7)
- "Locking the structure" – concentration is directed to the knee joints so that they "lock" in this position without any movement. The knees should feel as though they are being pushed in and out at the same time. This position will create "structure locking" in the feet as well and a strong "rooting" to the ground. This "locking" feeling is desired in the other body joints as well (elbows, shoulder girdle), and it will improve body strength and stability.

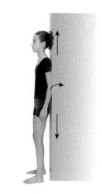

Figure 9.7 Organizing upper back, neck, and head position.

It must be emphasized that this position is not a natural posture but rather is a type of exercise that allows growth towards balanced posture. This is also the basis of the following exercise stages for improving body organization. Weakness and imprecise functioning of the basing energy impair overall body functioning, both in static situations and in movement. For this reason, in treating postural disorders it is recommended to devote the time needed to this initial stage of exercise.

Exercise to improve body alignment: standing without a wall

'Rooting' the feet

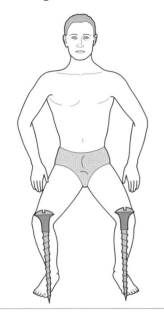

Figure 9.8 Rooting into the ground.

Like the foundation of a building, practicing foot rooting provides a strong basis on which balanced posture can be built while standing (Chia, 1993). In this exercise, patients visualize strong "roots" or "screws" coming out of their feet and gripping the ground (Fig. 9.8).

Balanced distribution of weight over the entire base of support on the foot (Fig. 9.5) is very important, and therefore, therapists should examine which areas experience more tension or pressure than others.

Lengthening the spinal column

After balancing the feet, one should slightly flex the knees, tilt the pelvis posteriorly and accentuate the lowering of the sacrum while stretching the head as though it were being pulled up by a string (Fig. 9.9). This position may create a feeling of lengthening the neck muscles and spinal column (traction). (Special traction exercises for the spinal column are detailed in Ch. 8).

Improving hip position

Hip joint stability depends on the condition of two other joints – the knees and the ankles. The critical point that makes good posture possible is a balanced positioning of the tibia bone in relation to the talus bone, which makes optimal stabilization possible for all body parts above the joint.

With a slight flexion of the knees, one should perform a slight lateral rotation of the knees. This action, which should be performed carefully and gently, will create a "spiral" movement downward, as if the feet were "screwed into" the ground (Chia, 1993) (Fig. 9.10). If for whatever reason there is a feeling of pain in the knee area, the rotational movement should be terminated or somewhat moderated.

Consistent practice of the training stages described above (with and without a wall) provides an essential basis for the coming exercise stages which are mostly based on various types of resistance with a partner.

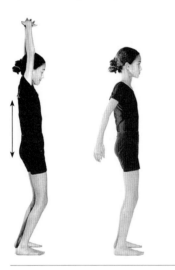

Figure 9.9 Lengthening the spinal column – while standing.

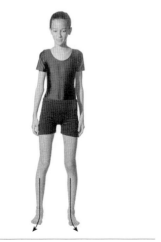

Figure 9.10 Consolidating foot grasp of the ground through slight rotational movement of the knees.

Resistance exercises: training to improve body rooting and posture muscle functioning

Exerting controlled pressure against the body with the assistance of a partner can strengthen basing in the ground and gradually activate the postural muscles. Using this technique consistently may be very effective in treating postural disorders and other limitations of the locomotor system.

After patients have stabilized themselves in standing (according to the principles described in the preceding stages), the therapist begins to push them gently and gradually, on various parts of their body and in different directions.

Patients should resist these pushes, and to succeed in remaining in place, they must learn to transfer this external force to the feet, which then grip the ground powerfully (Fig. 9.11).

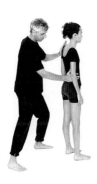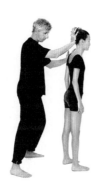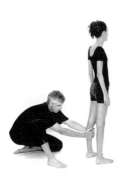

Figure 9.11 Resistance exercises.

As this type of training progresses, patients can relax quite well with no special effort. They must learn to feel the strength as it passes from the "pushed area". As they perceive and redirect it towards the ground, they will feel the resistant force that flows from the ground upward through the feet, so that they can resist the external push without "leaning" on the therapist (Chia, 1993). Exerting prolonged resistance of this type to various areas on the torso and spine will accustom them to correctly using the postural muscles in maintaining their balance and stability.

This technique also gives therapists the opportunity to feel functional asymmetries in different areas of the body and to identify them by evaluating patients' resistance power in these areas. Resistance should be applied consistently and for prolonged durations (5–10 s), and in different directions at the therapists' discretion. It is also advisable to use other starting points when performing this exercise (Fig. 9.12).

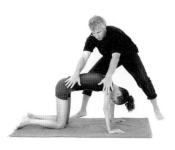
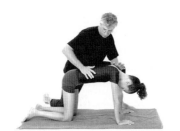
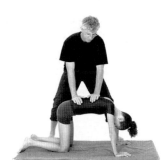
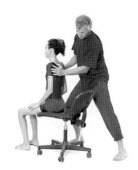
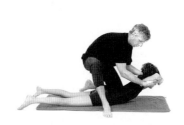

Figure 9.12A Working on balance and equilibrium in resistance exercises from different starting points.

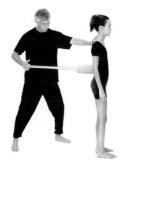
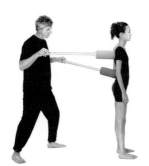
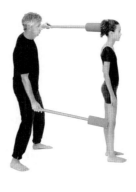
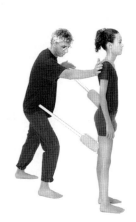

Figure 9.12B Use of "pillow polo" sticks as a means of exerting localized resistance in a number of areas simultaneously.

Theoretical aspects of resistance exercise techniques

Posture depends on normal functioning of the nervous system, which is capable of receiving information through the sensory organs, analyzing it, giving it meaning and guiding the movement patterns accordingly.

Underlying the research and practice of body organization theory is the assumption that adding structured sensory and movement activity helps the body to be more organized and directly affects neurological organization centers of the brain itself (Yakovlev & Lancours, 1967; Dennis, 1976).

The technique described earlier in this chapter enables therapists to diagnose functional imbalance according to the patients' physical responses to forces exerted on them. Correct and balanced responses require normal coordination, regulation of force and the ability to use body forces effectively. This is one of the examples of the subtle biological interrelationships through which peripheral sensory organs and central nerve cells communicate to create smooth, precise and automatic actions. Proper use of this mechanism requires to be learned.

Precision and perfection in muscular activity are acquired only through practice, and the technique described here is meant to meet this need, where remedial treatment is organized around these principles:

- Therapy should be aimed at strengthening patients' "rooting" ability in the ground, by organizing and aligning the body from the feet up
- Subjecting the body to external resistances exerted at varying degrees of strength and in different directions helps to activate postural muscles. The peripheral nervous system channels messages from the sensory organs and motor commands to the skeletal muscles. Constant and automatic feedback enables individuals to adjust their motor responses so that an accurate and fine motor control of muscle movements is achieved. This approach, which deals with the interrelationship between the nervous system and the musculoskeletal system, is founded upon numerous studies showing that brain functioning can be improved through motor movement training, and the reverse – that physical functioning can be improved by exposing the brain to stimuli (Kephart, 1960; Adams, 1971; Schmidt, 1988)
- As for posture organization, motor control is necessary to maintain normal positioning of the joints (in various starting positions and especially in standing). Such action requires high level body awareness and control, which is almost impossible without normal kinesthetic ability and coordination.

Gradual and consistent training may enable patients to develop motor control while maintaining the correct functional relationship between body limbs. Improved motor control combined with heightened physical awareness may in time bring about an improvement in movement and postural patterns.

The underlying assumption in this therapeutic approach places greater emphasis on "functional precision" of the movement system and less on strengthening specific muscles without considering overall functioning. For example, it may be possible to improve abdominal muscle strength but if these muscles are strengthened and activated incorrectly, the result may still be excessive lordosis in an erect stance.

The therapist's aim in practicing resistance exercises is to "direct" the patient to the proper activation of muscles for improved overall posture.

Other techniques for improving posture and body awareness

"Leading" exercises

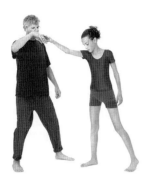

As noted, the ability to balance and stabilize the body in different starting positions is an essential prerequisite for normal functioning in both static and dynamic situations. The "leading exercise" technique can yield useful therapeutic results in the following areas:

- Dynamic balance
- Body organization and self and general spatial orientation (movement in different directions, at different rhythms and at different heights)
- Training to improve the feelings of movement (kinesthesis), combining work with eyes open and closed.

Sherington (1906) refers to kinesthesis as a "sixth sense" connected to that constant but unconscious sensory flow through body parts in movement (muscles, tendons, joints) (see Ch. 2). Kinesthesis facilitates continuous regulation and monitoring of movement, placement and tone, which is why it is so important for posture. "Leading" exercises have much to contribute in these areas.

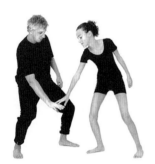

Manner of implementation

Stage 1: Therapists extend their hand forward. Patients place their hand lightly on the back of the therapists' hand. From this moment, they should maintain continuous contact.

Stage 2: Therapists begin to move their hand slowly in different directions and at different heights, and patients adjust themselves to these movements without breaking hand contact.

Leading exercises have many variations (Fig. 9.13)

- Movement in self spatial orientation at different heights
- Movement in general spatial orientation in different directions
- Movement with eyes closed, to work on kinesthesis
- Leading exercises using a stick
- Leading exercises using a skip rope.

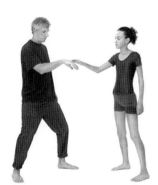

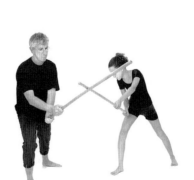
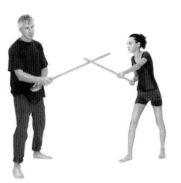

Figure 9.13 Variations of "leading" exercises with eyes open and closed.

"Raindrops" for locating tension points and improving body awareness

The aim of employing this technique is to help patients to "locate" and release tension points in their body. Localized "pressing" is used, on the assumption that touch helps to stimulate patients' awareness of various areas with heightened muscle tone in their body (Fig. 9.14).

Just as it is more effective for an outsider to edit a written text than it is for the author, in the therapeutic process, which is a kind of "editing", the therapist finds hidden, unknown tensions in the patient's body.

Manner of implementation

- Patient stands naturally with eyes closed
- Using one finger, the therapist presses different points on the patient's body, holding the pressure for a few seconds
- The patient directs his awareness to these areas and checks whether they are too tense.

Emphases in performance

- In order to maintain continuous contact with the patient, a new point should be pressed before a finger is removed from the previous point
- It is advisable to go over the following areas gradually: neck, shoulders, scapulae, both sides of the spinal column, thighs, calves, and feet.

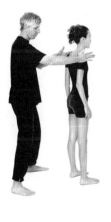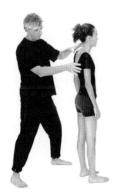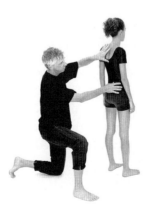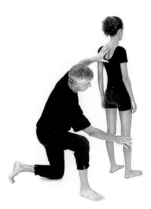

Figure 9.14 "Raindrops" in work on body awareness and locating tension points throughout the body.

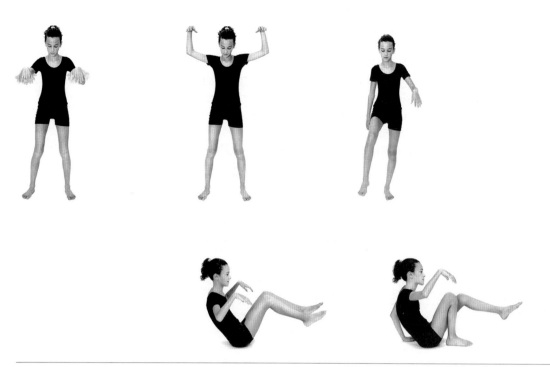

Figure 9.15 Variations in practicing the shaking out technique.

The "shaking out" technique for movement flow and muscle relaxation

This technique is especially effective for working on:

- Coordination – differentiated movement – regulation of force
- Movement flow
- Variations of static and dynamic balance
- Relaxation and reducing heightened muscle tone.

Manner of implementation Relaxing body joints while making "shaking out" movements from various starting points. Shaking out movements require a high level of motor control, and are characterized by a release of muscle tone, much like "shaking water" off one's hands. The technique can be performed in a number of variations (Fig. 9.15):

- Shaking out both arms while standing
- Shaking out right leg and left hand (work on coordination and balance)
- Shaking out arms and legs while seated
- Shaking out arms and legs while rolling forward and backward
- Shaking out the entire body while lying on the back.

Free movement within a structured framework

Free movement within a structured framework determined by the therapist makes it possible to act through self-listening and self-awareness, while actively investigating movement options from different starting points. This is one way to work on body image, self spatial orientation, cognitive ability in problem solving, etc.

During the exercise, patients create movement from within themselves without any guidance from the therapist. In this way, they expand their movement repertoire while internalizing functional ties between different body limbs. The format of this activity is not an "exercise" but rather a movement process that enables individuals to adapt their movements to personal feelings and to the limitations "imposed" upon them by the starting position.

The therapist creates the structured framework by determining a specific starting point. Within the limitations created by that starting point, patients should seek and find movement options within their own personal spatial orientation (examples of this type of process can be seen in Figs 9.16–9.22).

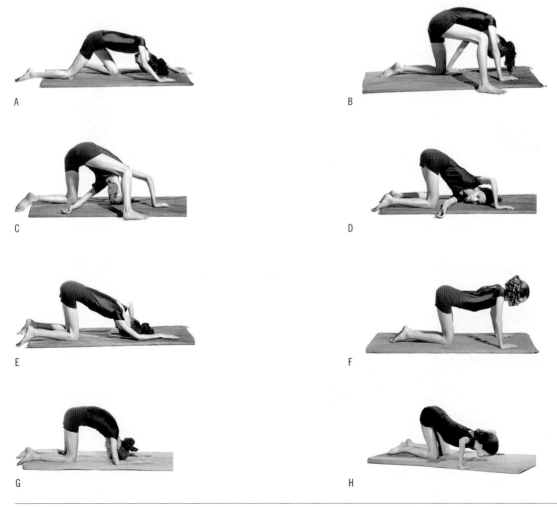

A

B

C

D

E

F

G

H

Figure 9.16 Possibilities for free movement from a hands-and-knees starting position.

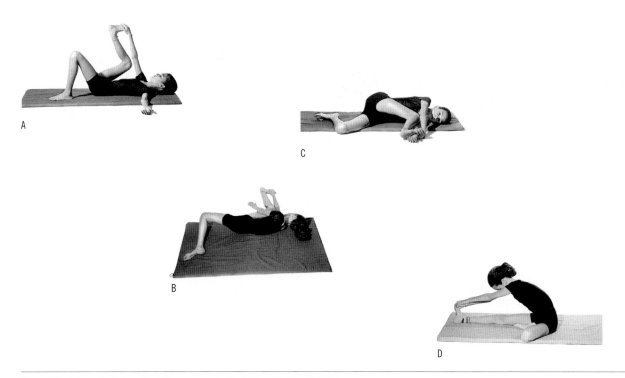

Figure 9.17 Lying on back, knees bent. Free movement with right hand holding right foot.

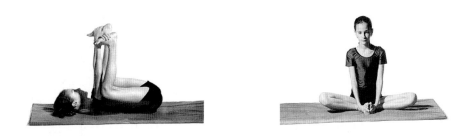

Figure 9.18 Free movement lying on back, with hands holding feet.

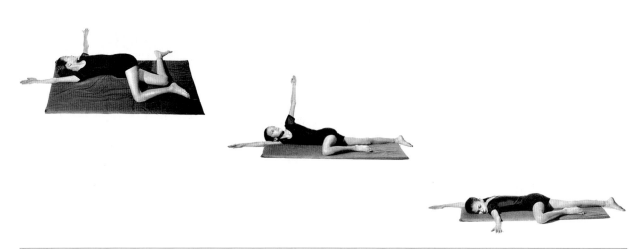

Figure 9.19 Free movement lying face down with right hand remaining straight forward.

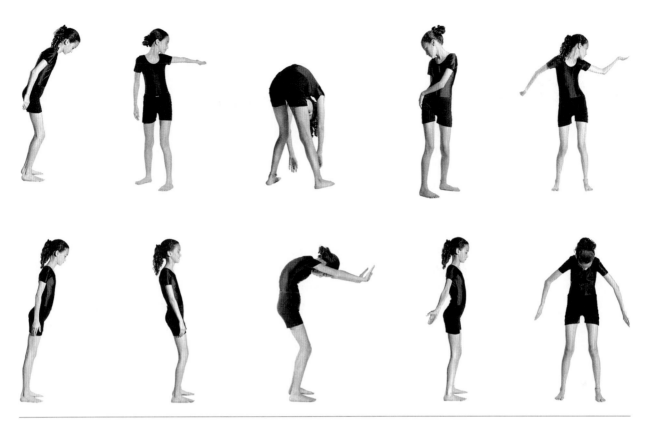

Figure 9.20 Free movement standing without moving feet (self-spatial orientation).

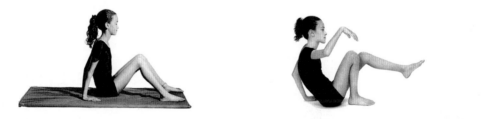

Figure 9.21 Free movement while sitting with opposite arm and leg.

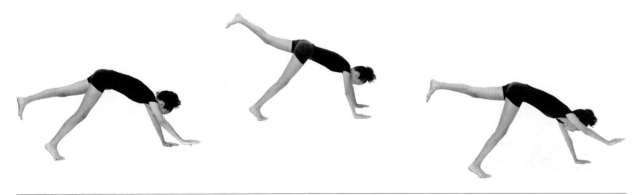

Figure 9.22 Free movement from a four-point stance with opposite arm and leg.

Manual guidance in postural exercises

Manipulative (manual) guidance makes use of kinesthetic perception and includes physical guidance or manipulation of the patient's body (Fig. 9.23). Touch may heighten awareness of specific movements by creating a supportive movement framework. This technique is especially effective for movements that require kinesthetic ability. The sensory feedback provided by the therapist by means of guiding touch may help patients to better understand the source of their errors, find solutions for them, and later improve their movement performance. Furthermore, the use of touch also provides a supportive framework that may help to gradually increase ranges of motion.

Emphases for implementation Care should be taken that touch in this context does not make patients passive; they must move their body within the supportive framework the therapist creates. In this way, patients can internalize the desired movement directions, so that the use of touch gradually decreases as patients progress.

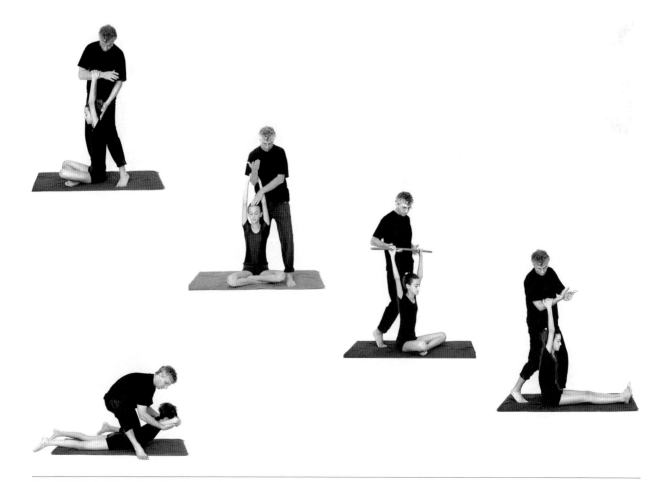

Figure 9.23 Manipulative guidance in various starting positions.

Using a stick for "contact and evasion" exercises

Activity with a stick encourages movement processes that develop several aspects of psychomotor functioning such as motor planning, reaction time, timing, balance, etc. Many variations can be devised for these exercises so that patients are exposed to different situations to which they must react in a suitable dynamic process.

The following examples refer to only two variations:

1. Contact in "defensive" stick exercises:

In this variation, patients should "protect" their body with a stick they hold with both hands, without moving their base of support in their feet. To do so, their movement reactions must follow the direction taken by the stick being wielded by the therapist (Fig. 9.24).

Emphases for implementation This exercise should be started very slowly, and supervised with care. The velocity of the movement should be increased gradually according to the patient's progress.

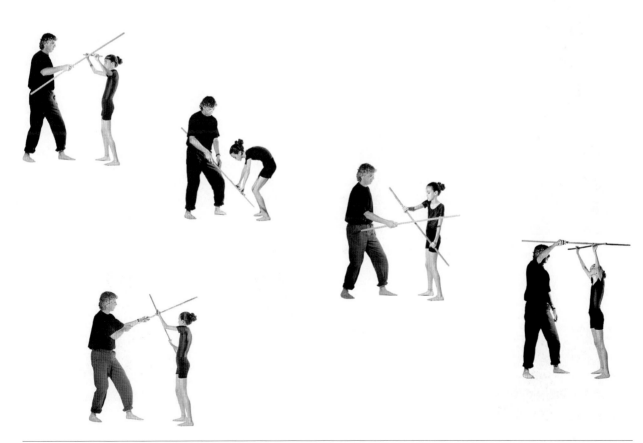

Figure 9.24 Contact in "defensive" exercises with a stick.

2. Evading the stick

This variation encourages work on self and general spatial orientation through continuous information processing (a cognitive component). Patients perceive and process information, and then produce an appropriate motor response.

Manner of implementation Patients stand on a pre-determined bounded surface (e.g., their personal mattress) and must avoid contact between the stick and their body, without leaving the marked area (Fig. 9.25).

Emphases for implementation

- There is a need to adjust the rhythm of the stick movements to patients' motor and cognitive abilities
- Two sticks can be used at the same time.

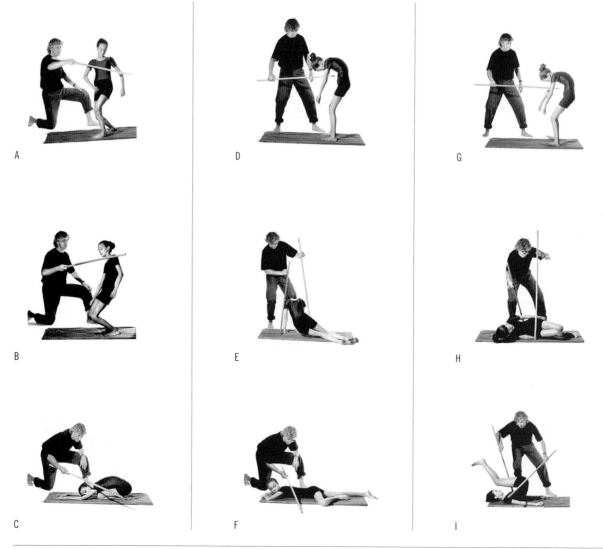

Figure 9.25 Evading the stick in self- and general spatial orientation.

Flexibility techniques for improving ranges of motion in treating postural disorders

Many postural disorders commonly found in the population are characterized by points of tension in various parts of the body and in reduced ranges of motion in the joints because of muscle shortening. Therefore, almost any treatment of postural disorders must integrate elements that emphasize work on flexibility, whether passively by the therapist or actively by means of exercises.

The essence of flexibility exercises is stretching active and passive connective tissues, among them muscles (which are a combination of active and passive tissue), and tendons, fascias, ligaments, and capsules (which are passive tissues) (Gur, 1998c).

Muscle length is a function of the strength ratio between antagonist muscles. Lack of balance between antagonist muscle groups changes the balance of forces acting on joints and affects their position. An integral part of treatment of postural disorders is bringing muscles to their appropriate length and strength to maintain optimal posture and functioning.

Methods of lengthening muscles are usually based on neurophysiological theories that have been tested and proven in the laboratory and clinic. The principle guiding them all is based on the assumption that to lengthen a muscle effectively, it must first be brought to a state of relaxation.

This section will deal with the neurophysiological basis underpinning several commonly used flexibility techniques, and will survey several guidelines for increasing flexibility properly and safely. These data are based on accepted kinesiological and biomechanical principles.

Factors causing shortened muscles and reduced ranges of motion

Connective tissues can become shorter, maintain their length or become longer. Muscle shortening in this context is attributable to several main causes:

- Prolonged fixation in a limited range (such as being in a cast or some other support apparatus)
- Lack of movement and one specific postural position for a long time
- Improper movement habits that are repeated over time.

The source of these factors is physical, but restricted ranges of motion and rigid movement patterns may also be caused by other factors, such as:

- Changes in muscle tone resulting from emotional stress (see Ch. 1)

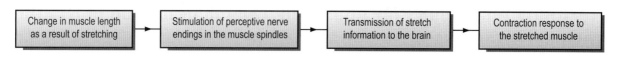

Figure 9.26 Action mechanism of muscle spindles.

- Impairment of kinesthetic ability that disrupts the transmission of information from kinesthetic receptors located in the joints to the central nervous system (see Ch. 2). This will also have an adverse effect on motor control and project onto movement patterns both in directed exercise and in daily functioning (ADL).

The neurophysiological basis for flexibility *(Gur, 1998a)* *

Aside from genetic dictates which determine general posture, muscle length and strength are the most important factors in overall functioning. While the genetic code affects mainly the osseous structure of the skeleton, the muscles (which function in a mutual balance between antagonist groups) affect body positions and joint functioning.

Muscle tissue has special qualities that permit:

- Contractility
- Extensibility
- Elasticity
- Ability to respond to a nervous stimulus from an electric, chemical or mechanic source.

As mentioned above, muscle tissue is a complex of passive and active tissues. In most of the structures connected to the locomotor system, such as muscles, tendons, ligaments, and fascias, there are perceptive bodies called proprioceptors. These contribute to control of muscle tone and movement coordination.

The main proprioceptors affecting functioning of the muscle system are (Figs 9.26, 9.27):

- Muscle spindles
- Golgi tendon organs.

Sensory organs perceive information in one way and transmit it by means of electric impulses to other parts of the central nervous system (CNS), where the information is decoded and processed as messages that are sent through the nervous system to the target organ or limb.

The proprioceptors mentioned (muscle spindles and Golgi organs) are sensitive to change in muscle length, movement speed, and the level of tension in the muscle.

*The material in this chapter about flexibility techniques is based on articles written by Dr Vardita Gur of the Zinman College at the Wingate Institute

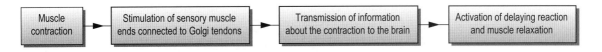

Figure 9.27 Action mechanism of Golgi tendon organs.

Muscle spindles

These proprioceptors, which are found mainly in the skeletal muscles, are highly sensitive to changes in muscle length and contain the ends of perceptive nerves. When a muscle lengthens, the perceptive nerve ends are stretched as well, and they report to the brain by means of the spinal cord that the stretch is approaching the limits of the muscle tissue range. In response – motor impulses are sent, and by means of movement neurons they cause the stretched muscle to contract (Fig. 9.26). This is the stretch reflex, which in essence is a protective mechanism to prevent the muscle from harmful stretching.

The stronger and faster the stretch is, or if it moves considerably greater than the existing range of motion, the stretch reflex will be stronger.

General relaxation and slow stretching that does not begin at the very end of the range, may raise the stimulation threshold of the muscle spindles, reduce its sensitivity to stretching, and thus moderate the stretch reflex (Basmajian, 1978). This aspect hints at the disadvantage inherent in flexibility methods that encourage rapid ballistic-type movements.

Golgi tendons

These proprioceptors are located in the tendon–muscle transfer point within the tendons and are especially sensitive to changes in muscle tension (Gur, 1998b). When the muscle contracts, the tendon fibers are stretched and exert pressure on the proprioceptive nerve endings connected to the Golgi tendons. These send out impulses to the spinal cord, which activates a delay response that moderates the muscle contraction (Fig. 9.27). This response, which causes the muscle to relax, occurs immediately as a reaction to a strong contraction, or after the tendon is stretched for 6–8 s.

This mechanism is very important in stretching techniques that entail the contraction of the stretched muscle as is done, for example, in the hold–relax technique described later in this chapter.

Accepted flexibility techniques for improving ranges of motion in treating postural disorders

Many options are available for maintaining or improving range of joint motion, whether by means of active and passive exercise or by means of a variety of treatment techniques that make use of touch (passive movement, massage, stretches performed by the therapist, etc.) (Kisner & Colby, 1985). From the various treatment methods, the following can be integrated easily and effectively into therapeutic work.

Active stretches

Active stretches entail contractions of the antagonist of the stretched muscle. For example, knee extension which is performed by the quadriceps, will cause the stretching of the hamstrings of the same leg (Fig. 9.28).

Passive stretches

Passive stretches do not actively involve the antagonist of the stretched muscle. For example, in a sitting position with the arms providing support, a forward leaning of the torso will cause a passive stretch of the hip extensors (hamstrings) (Fig. 9.29). The passive stretch facilitates relaxation of the stretched muscle, and may thus make the stretching process more effective.

Proprioceptive neuromuscular facilitation (PNF)

Reflexive activity is the basis of PNF stretch techniques. The assumption underlying the development of these techniques is that reducing muscle tension before and during the stretch is of great importance (Alter, 1988). In this context, extensive use is made mainly of two techniques:

Hold–Relax This technique is based on isometric voluntary contraction against resistance of the muscle that is to be lengthened, for example, stretching the pectoral muscles as shown in Figure 9.30.

Stage 1: Pushing the ground to create resistance for the muscle for 6–8 s
Stage 2: Relaxation
Stage 3: Extended stretch of 10–15 s.

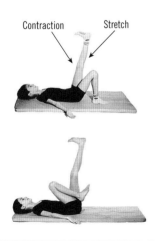

Figure 9.28 Active stretching of the hamstrings.

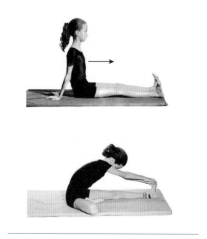

Figure 9.29 Passive stretching of the hamstrings.

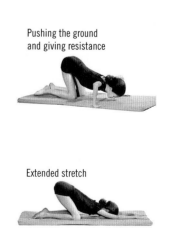

Figure 9.30 Stretching the pectoral muscles using the hold–relax technique.

Reciprocal innervation This technique is based on isometric contraction against resistance created by the antagonist to the stretched muscle. Here, use is made of the principle that muscle contraction will cause relaxation of the antagonist muscle, for example, when lower back muscles are stretched after contracting abdominal muscles, as illustrated in Figure 9.31.

Stage 1: Contraction of abdominal muscles by pressing the knees towards the chest for 6–8 s

Stage 2: Relaxation

Stage 3: Extended stretching of the lower back muscles for 10–15 s, by passively bringing the knees closer to the chest (using hands).

The techniques described here can be performed both independently (by patients creating their own resistance against a wall or the ground, or by pressing limbs against one another) and with the assistance of a partner or the therapist. In each approach, it is important to ensure gradual, balanced work and to avoid strong or overly long stretches.

In this vein, a number of important aspects should be mentioned about working to make muscles flexible (Gur, 1998b):

1. Isolation of the targeted muscles from other tissues.
2. The starting position should be comfortable for the patient without overloading any joint.
3. Stretching movements are more effective when the muscle is passive and tone is low.
4. To prevent damage, the exercises should be graded according to three factors:
   - Duration of stretch
   - Range of stretch
   - Speed of stretch.
5. In stretching muscles that cross two joints (such as the hamstrings, which go over the hip and the knee), it is best to begin working on each joint separately, and only afterwards on both at the same time.
6. The rhythm of exercises to improve flexibility should be slow and controlled, integrating a static hold at the end of the stretch range (for 4–8 s).
7. It is recommended to perform stretch and flexibility exercises after a light warm-up that raises body temperature slightly.
8. While performing stretches, sharp or excessive pain should be avoided. However, it should be kept in mind that stretching, whose main goal is mutation of soft tissue length, may cause a certain amount of discomfort.

In general, it can be said that gradual and controlled exercises of a few minutes a day is safer and more effective than heavy exercising once or twice a week.

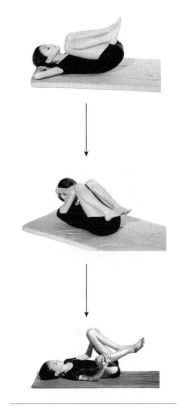

Figure 9.31 Stretching lower back muscles using the reciprocal innervation technique.

CHAPTER 10

Hydrotherapy in the treatment of postural disorders

Hydrotherapy is rapidly gaining acceptance today as a physical therapy and rehabilitation treatment. The main reason for its popularity lies in the special qualities of water (buoyancy, resistance, and heat) (Bergman & Hutzler, 1996). This chapter will discuss several therapeutic benefits of activity in water, and will also mention contraindications in the therapy process.

In this vein, it is worth re-examining the almost universal dictum that "swimming is a healthy activity". This belief tends to ignore the swimmer's limitations and the risks the activity entails.

Swimming is not necessarily healthy and in terms of treatment, if it is not adapted to patient's special needs, it may even be harmful (Solberg, 1995).

Often, orthopedists refer children for therapy in words to this effect: "The above patient has a postural disorder – swimming is recommended." This recommendation usually does not include any reference to the essence of the disorder any contraindications in treating it. According to this approach, anyone who passes a short basic swimming course can act as a hydrotherapist for children with postural disorders. However, treating these children is a complex process because of the limitless variations these disorders can assume. Therapists must deal with the complexity of the problem, and on the basis of an initial diagnosis, construct an activity program adapted specifically to the children's needs. This process requires much more than learning how to swim, and therefore by its very definition, the therapeutic technique is not "swimming" but "water adapted activity". According to this model, it may very well be that therapists choose to teach children a special swim style that does not appear in any conventional book on learning to swim.

The following are examples of a few disorders that require extra caution when using hydrotherapy

- In treating lordosis, the breaststroke is contraindicated because of the tendency to increase lumbar lordosis in the swimming movement (Fig. 10.1). This swimming style is also not recommended in cases of excessive cervical lordosis, heightened muscle tone in the erector spinae of the cervical spine, and structural pathologies such as spondylolysis and spondylolisthesis

- In treating scoliosis, the swimming style must be specifically adapted to the direction of the spinal deviation. This requires great expertise and must be done only by professionals in the field. If therapists choose to use only symmetrical movements (for overall physical exercise), it is recommended to concentrate on the classic backstroke

- In cases of disorders of the hip, knee and ankle joints, therapists must also take the diagnostic data into consideration (see Ch. 5). For example, the breast stroke is recommended for treating medial rotation of the lower extremities because it encourages the opposite movement (lateral rotation) in the hip joints. In the opposite condition, where the problem is characterized by a toe-out position, the freestyle (crawl) is recommended because it encourages medial rotation of the legs

- In certain conditions, such as Marfan's syndrome, which is characterized by over-flexibility of the joints, patients should be assigned a personal style that integrates arm movements characteristic of the breaststroke style and leg movements typical of the crawl. In this case, the regulation breaststroke is contraindicated because it increases ranges of hip joint movement and creates unwanted tension in the medial aspect of the knee joints (Fig. 10.1). Ignoring this information will cause the patient more harm than good.

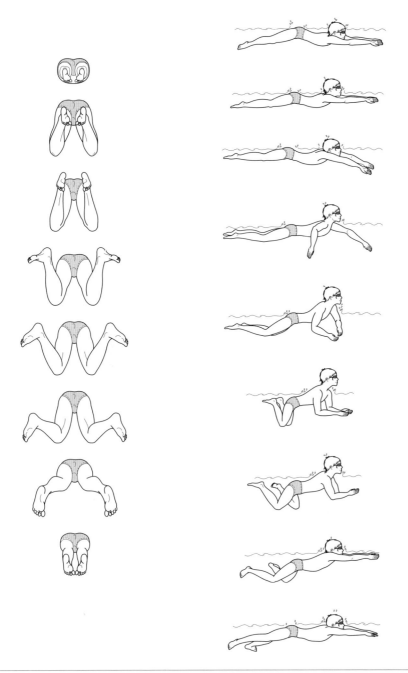

Figure 10.1 Swimming the breaststroke: Posterior and lateral views.

As these examples indicate, in treating postural disorders, swimming alone is not enough. Attention must be paid to information about the problem in order to determine the proper type of activity. Only in this way can treatment engender real improvement and even more importantly, avoid injury. Swimming has many benefits, but therapists must try to avoid adopting prepackaged programs that appear in the literature, and use their professional discretion in the therapeutic process.

Adapted water activity for postural disorders

In terms of indications for using hydrotherapy for postural disorders, a clear distinction should be made between physical medical indications and therapeutic sport indications (Snir, 1996).

Medical indications

Because of the special qualities of water, hydrotherapy is especially suitable for conditions that are vulnerable to injury from weight-bearing loads, such as idiopathic scoliosis, rehabilitation after back surgery, etc. In such cases, water increases relaxation, maintains – and even increases – ranges of joint motion, and when needed, strengthens various muscles without creating vertical loads on body joints, especially on the spinal column.

Many postural disorders are characterized by heightened muscle tone with resulting movement restrictions. Water (at a comfortable temperature) may help to bring the muscular system to a state of relaxation, and thus encourage freer movement of the problematic area. Relaxation of this type can help children to attain normal muscle tone, and encourage broader ranges of motion. In general, the ability to relax combined with reduced effects of gravity improve movement potential in cases of children with a variety of disabilities, among them postural disorders.

Therapeutic sport indications

Water activity adheres to the principles of therapeutic sport. Special emphasis is placed on the gradual transition from "exercises" defined as the "therapeutic component" to active physical and recreational activity (learning to swim).

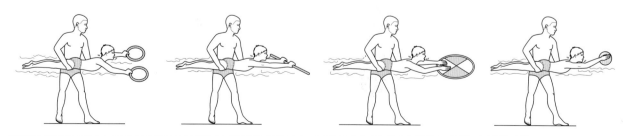

Figure 10.2 Use of various types of apparatus in water activities.

In planning a therapy and rehabilitation program in water, a number of factors should be kept in mind (Bergman & Hutzler, 1996):

- *Water depth*: Buoyancy support increases as large parts of the body are submerged in water, therefore it is recommended to execute some of the exercises for the lower part of the body in deeper water first and then progress gradually to shallow water. On the other hand, maximal resistance will be attained when the entire body is submerged in water, which is important when performing exercises to strengthen the upper part of the body and upper extremities

- *Movement speed and range of motion*: Movement speed has a significant effect on water resistance: a small increase in speed increases resistance considerably. Similarly, increasing patients' range of motion also raises the level of difficulty. For these reasons, it is advisable that patients begin activities slowly and with a small range of motion, then gradually increase both speed and range. Usually improper movement patterns indicate that patients are working beyond their ability in terms of range of motion or speed

- *Patients' position*: Patients' positions during their water activity should be determined by diagnostic results and by the characteristics of the disorder. Activity may include a variety of starting positions such as sitting, standing, lying face down, lying on back, etc. Each position has kinesiological implications for the musculoskeletal system, which is why it is important to adapt the recommended swimming style to the various postural disorders

- *Closed kinematic chain and open kinematic chain*: In designing a hydrotherapy program, it is possible to control the intensity of the gravity load using buoyancy as a resistive force. A joint that moves against a constant resistance source, such as the ground, creates a closed kinematic chain. In this way, exercises performed while standing in shallow water are usually similar to closed kinematic chain exercises, even though the load on the joint is smaller (than on land) because of the opposing force of buoyancy. On the other hand, exercises in deep water are usually referred to as open kinematic chain exercises – exercises that are performed horizontally (like swimming). Various resistive apparatus tend to "close" a kinematic chain.

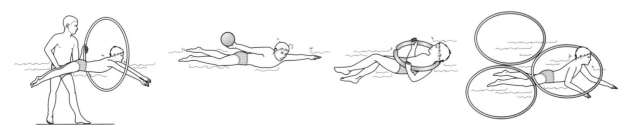

Figure 10.2 (*continued*).

The decision whether to use closed or open kinematic chain exercises is left to the discretion of the therapists, who should base their decisions on the nature of the problem and the aims of the therapy.

Water activity as a means of therapeutic intervention for postural disorders concentrates on a number of major aspects (Solberg, 1995) as noted below.

Work on body awareness and body image

How people refer to the world around them depends on their body image. If they are not completely aware of their bodies, any action requiring such awareness will be flawed. Perceptions of the "self" are embedded in relationships with self and general spatial orientation, where the central reference point is the body. Many children with postural disorders have difficulty in this respect because of various asymmetries in their body position, and therefore, among other things, their movement learning is imperfect and they adopt erroneous movement patterns. Activity in water allows patients to experience new movement options, and exercising in self- and general spatial orientation in water also contributes to enhancing body awareness.

Apparatus such as skip ropes, hoops and balls are possible aids that allow children to raise their awareness about their own body and objects around them (Fig. 10.2). This aspect is especially important in cases of "new" limitations, such as injuries to the spinal column and physical disabilities resulting from accidents.

Improving general body system functioning

1. Respiratory system: The very act of being submerged in the water entails constant pressure on the chest and lungs, which has a positive effect on respiratory system functioning. Water activity raises patients' awareness of the breathing process, including its rhythm and duration (Bergman & Hutzler, 1996). Furthermore, water activity also facilitates work to improve cardiopulmonary endurance (by means of endurance exercises in water).

2. Improving ranges of joint motion by active and passive stretches: This is important mainly in cases of orthopedic problems (before and after surgery). Water activity may help patients to return to regular independent functioning.

3. Improving muscle strength and endurance is also an important component for improving functioning. Water creates resistance to active movement on all planes, and thus facilitates exercise and practice for muscles and joints in a wide array of implementation angles. Exercise can be performed in movements involving the entire body (swimming, walking) or movements isolating specific limbs by holding onto the wall for support (Bergman & Hutzler, 1996).

4. Neuromuscular functioning, mainly for improving coordination and balance: Water activity offers an array of means of working on disabilities characteristic of many postural disorders. The advantage of water activity in these cases lies in the slowing down of various movement stages (because of water resistance), thus producing highly effective "learning conditions".

Coordination problems and difficulties in maintaining balance can be treated in water by practicing variations of transitions from one physical position to another, changing movement direction, changing rhythm (slow, fast, stop), changing style while advancing, etc. Such exercising will also affect patients' awareness of the kinesthetic feedback they receive during the activity.

These are some examples of exercises for improving balance

- Transition from standing in water to floating on stomach and back to standing
- Transition from floating on stomach to floating on back
- Advancing while swimming the sidestroke and changing the direction of movement from side to side
- Swimming in circles from right to left
- Swimming a "slalom" between floats
- Swimming forward, stopping in place and swimming backward
- Regular walking in water
- Walking on toes
- Walking on heels
- Walking heel to toe
- Walking sideways – to the right and to the left
- Moving forward in two-leg jumps in shallow water
- Moving forward in one-leg hops in shallow water
- "Stepping leaps" with arm–leg coordination, in water at hip or chest height
- Standing in place on one leg and maintaining body balance using arm motions (therapists can "stir up" the water around the patients and create waves to raise the level of difficulty for maintaining body balance).

Exercises of this sort have many possible variations. Over time, training will lead to better mastery of the transitions between body positions and to improved balance ability, coordination and body organization in both personal and general space. This improvement may also be reflected in the children's functioning outside of water.

Improvement in affective (emotional) functioning

Activity offering pleasure and a feeling of "success" is highly important for children with disabilities (both affective and physical). Water activity allows children with physical disabilities to shed all the auxiliary aids they need for regular land-based activity (walkers, support braces for the spine, etc.) and to behave freely in the water. The new physical abilities they reveal in the water will be an experience of success and satisfaction that will reinforce their self confidence and self esteem.

Principles for planning a hydrotherapy program for children with postural disorders

The principles presented here are based on additional aspects that are detailed in Chapter 14. Building a therapeutic program must personally suit the children's needs as determined by an initial diagnosis that includes cognitive, affective, social, and physical condition, as well as motor abilities in water and outside it (see Ch. 7).

- Each meeting should include two components:
  a. A therapeutic component – specific exercises for the type of problem or disability (exercises for strength and flexibility, different manners of advancing in water, breathing exercises, etc.).
  b. Play and enjoyment – this will enhance motivation, perseverance and patient–therapist ties (ball games, use of various apparatus, diving games, etc.). In this model, the initial activity emphasis is on the affective side. Safe and enjoyable activity in this domain will usually heighten motivation and prepare the groundwork for success in future treatment.

- Every few months it is advisable to conduct comprehensive postural tests outside of the water to monitor progress and to set treatment aims for continuation. It should be remembered that in most cases, postural disorders are dynamic. They may improve or they may worsen, but they usually do not remain unchanged. Therapists must be aware of these changes and adapt themselves to the children's condition.

To illustrate what has been presented up to this point, the following therapeutic program is presented as an example of dealing with kyphosis, a common postural disorder.

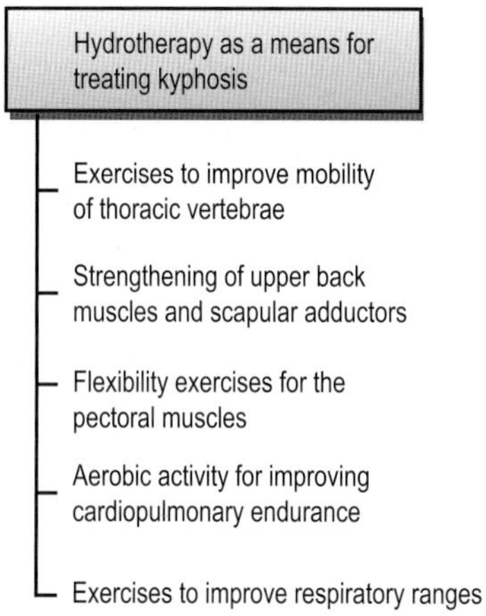

Treating kyphosis

Main aspects of the disorder

Kyphosis is marked by an exaggerated arch in the thoracic vertebrae and a tendency of the shoulders and head to tilt forward (see Ch. 3). Other common characteristics are possible shortening of the pectoral muscles, weakness in the upper back area and sometimes increased cervical lordosis. Breathing may also be short and shallow, and body awareness weak.

In light of the above, hydrotherapy treatment should concentrate on a number of aspects (Fig. 10.3):

Hydrotherapy as a means for treating kyphosis

- Exercises to improve mobility of thoracic vertebrae

- Strengthening of upper back muscles and scapular adductors

- Flexibility exercises for the pectoral muscles

- Aerobic activity for improving cardiopulmonary endurance

- Exercises to improve respiratory ranges

Figure 10.3 Main aspects of hydrotherapeutic treatment of kyphosis.

- Exercises to stretch and lengthen pectoral muscles
- Strengthening upper back muscles, mainly the scapular adductors
- Breathing exercise to increase range of respiration (mainly inhalation)
- Aerobic activity to improve cardiopulmonary endurance
- Practice to improve thoracic vertebrae mobility (T1–T12)
- Awareness and relaxation exercises.

Recommended exercises for kyphosis

The list of exercises proposed here is an example of gradual training in water for meeting special needs:

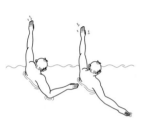

1. Standing in water up to shoulder height – actively stretching arms with circular movements up and backward.

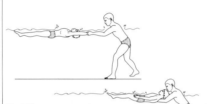

2. Therapist executes passive stretches while patient lies motionless on back, arms straight and stretched backward (behind the head).

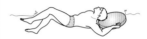

3. Lying on the back holding a board with arms straight backwards – making leg movements as in breaststroke or crawl; maintaining straight body position without raising head forward (and making sure pelvis does not sink).

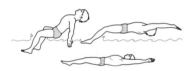

4. Back push off – holding side of pool with hands and pushing back hard while stretching the body.

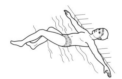

5. Holding side of pool with both stretched hands, back to wall and doing cycling movements with legs (when performed for extended periods this is also an endurance exercise that also stretches pectoral muscles with arms to the sides).

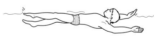

6. Swimming in the classical backstroke style – circular arm movements near the center of body

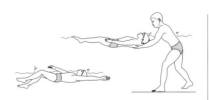

7. Back crawl – full movement with arms straight, near central axis of body. Occasionally therapist should provide support between the scapulae.

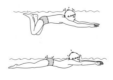

8. Forward gliding – pushing the wall with legs and stretching arms forward while lowering head and exhaling in the water.

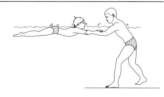

9. Lying floating on the stomach, arms straight and supported by the therapist – legs kicking as in the crawl style combined with exhaling in the water.

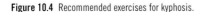

Figure 10.4 Recommended exercises for kyphosis.

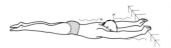

10. Floating on the stomach, hands straight forward and grasping the rim of the pool – legs kicking as in the crawl while exhaling in the water.

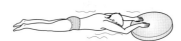

11. Swimming on the stomach while holding a board with body straight and tensed – legs movement as in breaststroke or crawl.

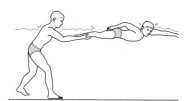

12. Swimming the freestyle (crawl) with the therapist holding the patient's legs under water and creating light resistance.

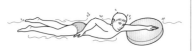

13. Swimming freestyle with one hand, while the other is holding a float board.

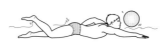

14. Pushing a ball while swimming the crawl.

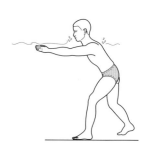

15. Walking forward in water up to the shoulders while strongly pulling the water from front backwards without removing arms from the water.

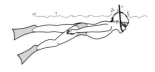

16. Practicing breathing in the water using a snorkel and fins.

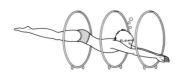

17. Diving from a sitting position on the pool lip, passing through hoops weighted in the water.

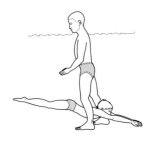

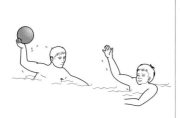

18. Passing a ball – in deep water.

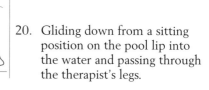

19. Relaxing while floating on the back, taking deep breaths – with therapist supporting the body.

20. Gliding down from a sitting position on the pool lip into the water and passing through the therapist's legs.

Figure 10.4 (continued).

The exercises presented in this program are for illustration only, and can be adapted, developed and altered as long as water safety rules and accepted kinesiological principles are adhered to. At the same time, as mentioned, an important part of treating postural disorders entails changing existing movement patterns and intensive work on body awareness. For this reason, it is recommended to integrate water activity with regular remedial exercise outside the water, to attain optimal results.

Summary

One of the main aims of this chapter is to encourage therapists to use their discretion in choosing rehabilitative activity in water. To this end, several main aspects have been reviewed, including the advantages of water activity as a therapeutic intervention for postural problems and the principles for building a hydrotherapy treatment program.

Postural disorders are complex, as is the nature of the treatment planned for each problem. Treatment of kyphosis, as presented in this chapter, is a specific example of how to construct an activity program for postural disorders.

CHAPTER 11

Auxiliary equipment for adapted physical activity

In order to design a therapeutic program properly, therapists must understand the nature of the disorder they are treating and correctly analyze the functional–motor difficulties it engenders. This is the basis on which therapists should introduce varied and interesting activities to improve these functions.

This chapter will deal with ways of creatively using auxiliary aids during the treatment of postural disorders on the assumption that the proper use of apparatus and equipment may help to stimulate cognitive, affective, and physical developmental processes.

Creative use of equipment in treatment

Over the years, the ability of children to plan or create organized patterns progresses along a movement continuum. Improvement on this continuum can be observed in their expanding repertoire of physical abilities and in their normal movement and postural patterns.

Maturation of the central nervous system is a prerequisite for normal functioning, but rich motor exposure and appropriate practice also play an important role in the process of acquiring a wide array of skills.

Numerous models have been developed for the improvement of motor functioning. The comprehensive treatment approach advocated in this book relies on two eminent models.

The "underlying abilities" model

According to the underlying abilities approach, basic motor abilities are an indispensable prerequisite for success in various skills of daily functioning; for example, coordination and balance are the basis for normal walking. These abilities are indispensable for optimal functioning. Moreover, they are included or integrated in the required skill and therefore treatment techniques that make use of this model emphasize work on movement components.

The "working on the whole" model

This therapeutic model, in contrast, is based on the idea that treatment should emphasize activities that include the underlying abilities, and not work on developing them separately. In other words, even though the underlying abilities are included and integrated in the required skills, there is also a reverse effect – when the whole skill is activated, underlying abilities will necessarily be involved in them. Therefore, according to this approach, full activation of the inclusive whole will contribute to the improvement of the components.

This would seem to be one of the differences between the adapted physical activity approach and other treatment techniques. While in paramedical treatment therapists usually emphasize working on posture components (specific exercises for stretching and strengthening muscles); the adapted physical activity approach also emphasizes work on whole skills as a means of treating these components.

The learning process in this approach is active. For example, if the therapist wants a child to perform elbow extension, it is possible to design a task such as hammering a nail or shooting a ball at a basket. After the child has performed arm extension, the therapist can call his attention to the desired result (extension of the elbow joint) so that the child can implement it in other situations as well (transference).

The recommended way of treating children with postural disorders combines both models.

Another important aspect of this integrative approach is the child's enjoyment of the treatment process. Success and an enjoyable feeling in the activities constitute important bases for motivating children to continue working. The basic assumption is that if children enjoy an activity, they will be more motivated to carry on with it and make the effort it requires of them. This means that one of the important challenges facing therapists is finding ways to activate children in a manner that appeals to their interests and personality and that are, at the same time, relevant to the treatment aims.

An example illustrating this approach entails two types of exercises for strengthening back muscles (see Fig. 11.1).

Both exercises are equally effective in attaining the goal – strengthening the back muscles – but they differ in both manner and approach. In Exercise A, the patient concentrates on the effort and at times performs the exercise with a feeling of discomfort mixed with boredom. In Exercise B, in contrast, the child is given an interesting and challenging task that both helps to strengthen the back and impart a feeling of enjoyment. In this situation, the child will concentrate less on the difficulty and effort, and more on the experience itself.

As noted, it is recommended to use both methods, that is, "sterile" more precise drills together with tasks that utilize adapted apparatus and place greater emphasis on the children's interests, motivation, consideration of their personality, and materials that appeal to them (see Fig. 11.2).

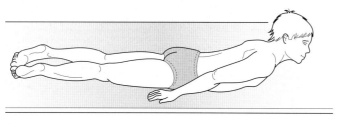

A

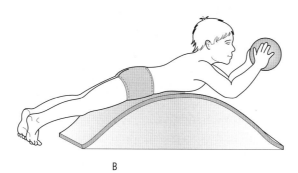

B

Figure 11.1 (A,B) Exercises to strengthen back muscles.

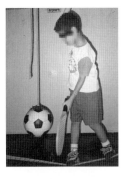

Differentiation of movement and regulation of force using hanging ropes and racquet.

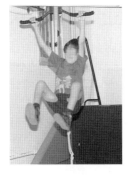

Working with an omega.

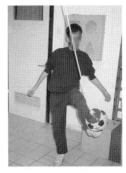

Kicking a hanging ball for work on timing and coordination.

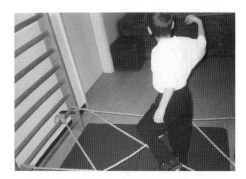

Going through an obstacle course to improve movement planning and spatial orientation.

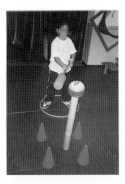

Crossing the midline and visuomotor coordination with pillow-polo poles.

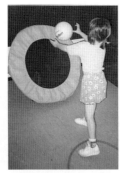

Exercise in passing and catching using a trampoline and ball.

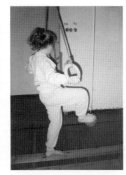

Static balance and movement timing on a bench.

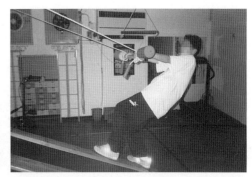

Simulation of surfing using an inclined bench.

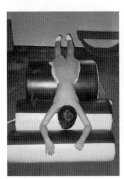

Passive movement on three inclined rollers.

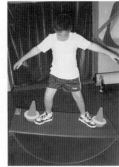

Balance exercise on rolling surface.

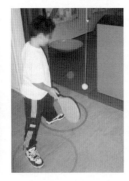

Improving racquet skills with hanging ball.

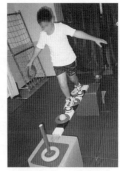

Static and dynamic balance on a balance bar.

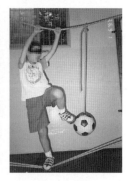

Body organization with hanging ropes and ball.

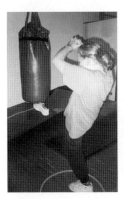

Kicking a punching bag to improve balance and coordination

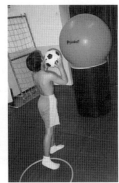

Practicing passing and catching using a physiotherapy ball and roll.

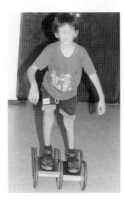

Riding a Pedalo to improve motor control and balance.

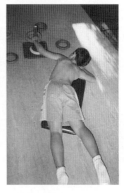

Strengthening back and shoulder girdle in activity with scooter.

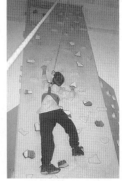

Climbing wall to nurture self confidence and work on movement planning.

Figure 11.2 Adapted use of equipment during treatment.

CHAPTER 12

Movement and postural development in early childhood: principles and applications

The first years of children's lives are marked by changes in motor and physical development. The movement activity to which children are exposed during these years plays a predominant role in shaping their abilities in the future. Children observe their limbs, feel them and move them in their personal and general space. As mastery of their body becomes more refined, their increasing motor control allows them to gradually acquire skills such as grasping, throwing and catching a ball, passing a ball, crawling and walking, by using the developing abilities of balance, coordination, regulation of force, kinesthesis, etc.

The many movements that children attempt make them function more efficiently and improve their ability to plan and differentiate movements, perceive direction and develop spatial orientation. All of these skills contribute to molding the children's posture and facilitating their normal physical development.

However, a lack of awareness of these skills may impair children's movement and posture development. Many children who do not receive sufficient exposure to movement activity experience difficulties stemming from motor deficiencies. In other cases, various posture disorders develop because the children remain in certain body positions for long periods of time or have faulty movement habits.

Normal development in children is a mix of both genetic inherited and environmental factors. Despite significant genetic effects on children's posture and development, environmental elements are also of great significance. Parents and professionals who come in contact with children in early childhood should be keenly aware that all issues pertaining to physical activity may be important for optimal development.

Such awareness naturally raises questions:

- Should an infant sleep on the back or the belly?
- How should children be encouraged to sit?
- Should children be helped in walking or should they attempt it themselves?
- How can children be activated so as to improve their overall physical strength?

This chapter will survey important aspects of movement and postural development in early childhood as a means of preventing, as much as possible, the appearance of disorders at a later age.

Common developmental characteristics of early childhood

Birth–2 years old

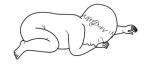

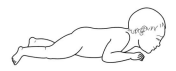

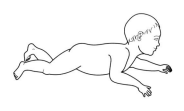

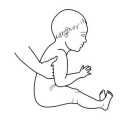

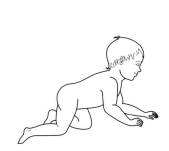

This period is characterized by continuous development from reflexive involuntary activity to more controlled and organized movement. Infant motor development includes several milestones, such as head-raising, turning over, crawling, sitting, standing and walking.

These stages of infant motor development during the first year contribute both to posture (general strengthening and gradual development of the spinal curves), and to motor abilities (gross motor development as well as providing an important functional basis for fine motor activity). Basic motor patterns appear during the initial developmental period in a defined and predictable sequence. Keeping this in mind, it is important to review a number of universal principles of motor development which become evident in some common patterns (Yazdi-Ugav, 1995).

Cephalocaudal direction

Gross motor development begins from the top down, towards the legs. In this process, motor control and mastery develop and take shape first in the head area (strength of the neck muscles), then moves down to the upper torso and upper extremities, and gradually reaches the lower torso and lower extremities (Yazdi-Ugav, 1995).

In this way, infants experience a number of developmental milestones, such as raising their head while lying on their belly, rising to a leaning position on forearms and elbows, sitting, crawling, standing and walking (Fig. 12.1).

Incomplete patterns of cephalocaudal direction may be reflected in developmental retardation, and later in heavy and clumsy movements.

Proximal–distal coordination

The muscles closer to the midline of the body become functionally capable in terms of coordination and motor control faster than the muscles further away from the midline. This developmental pattern

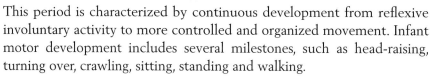

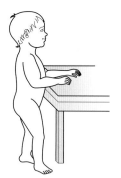

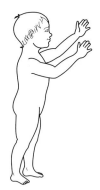

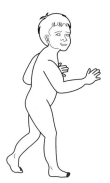

Figure 12.1 Milestones in motor development: First year.

underlines the functional ties between gross and fine motor activity where, for example, the strength of the large muscle groups in the shoulder girdle provides the stability necessary for the hands and fingers to perform the fine motor manipulations required for writing, cutting, buttoning, etc.

What these facts emphasize is the body's need for activity to strengthen large muscle groups that contribute to body stability in daily functioning.

Motor behavior is affected by the infant's neurological functioning

Neural development is reflected in progress from simple, massive and reflexive movements to fine, integrative movement.

Many of the reflexive movements that develop after birth serve as the basis for the development of movement patterns that are later controlled by the higher control centers in the brain (Yazdi-Ugav, 1995). It should be remembered that motor development is dependent in great part on the rate of the infant's neurological maturation, and this process cannot by hastened by specific training.

Attempts to speed up natural processes may also cause damage. For example, encouraging children to stand or walk before these activities occur naturally can create overload on the hip or knee joints and impair optimal development (the "first child syndrome").

At the same time, although some of the infant's neuromuscular responses are reflexive in nature, most are voluntary and learned, and influenced by environmental factors and previous experience. Thus, as infants progress in their physical development, the ratio between involuntary and voluntary responses is modified, as reflexes slowly disappear, and controlled coordinative movements develop.

This accounts for the importance of exposing children to rich motor stimulation (by forming a stimulating environment) that encourages them to act, strengthens them and also ensures that they will not be deficient in the array of movements in their arsenal. Apart from improving children's movement patterns, this approach may also have a positive emotional side-effect of improving their self confidence and self esteem (Fig. 12.2).

Ages 2–4

This period in children's lives is characterized by the refinement of existing motor functions, together with the acquisition of new skills such as running, climbing, and jumping. Fine motor coordination also improves gradually, allowing children to better control their movements, even the fine movements performed by small muscle groups.

Physically, this is a stage of constant physical body growth. Skeletal growth is relatively fast, and the bones are mainly cartilaginous and soft. Muscular system development is concentrated predominantly in the large muscle groups, and the spinal curves continue to develop slowly.

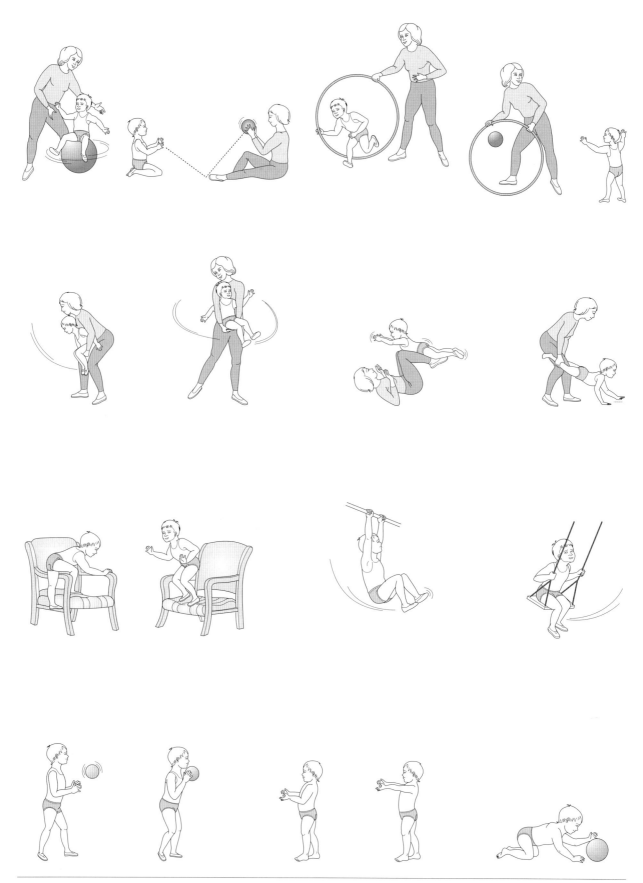

Figure 12.2 Psychomotor exposure during various developmental periods of early childhood. The emphasis in the examples presented is on simple and available motor activities that can be performed in the family setting (home, yard, or playground), and which may contribute to the child's normal development both physically and emotionally. The emphasis in these activities is more on motor experience and pleasure, and less on the final results of the movement.

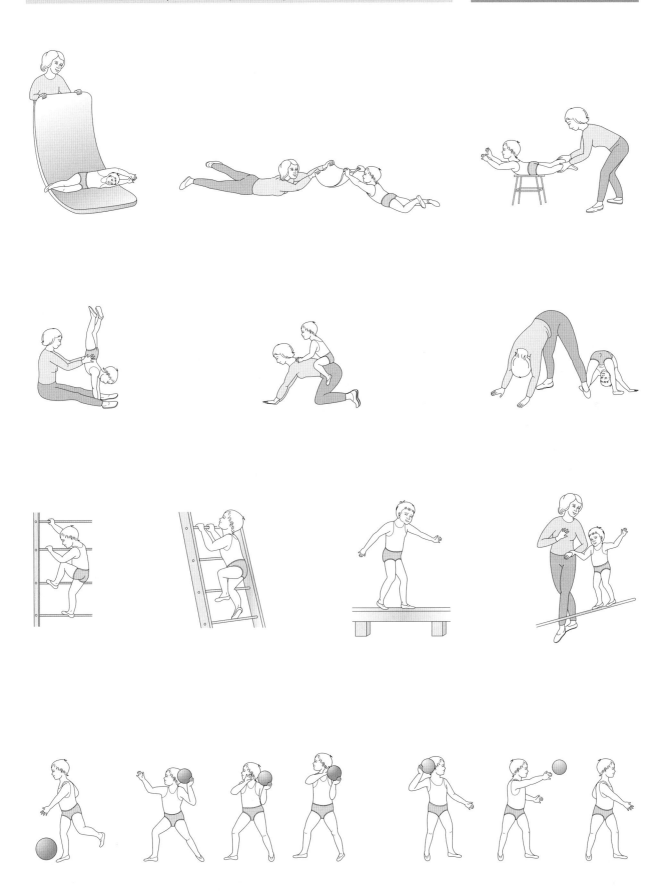

Figure 12.2 (*continued*).

Orthopedic aspects and common postural disorders in early childhood: diagnosis, prevention, and treatment

The development of disorders in the lower extremities is quite common in early childhood (see also Ch. 5). These disorders may develop as the result of an inborn defect, genetic factors or environmental factors (movement habits, motor deficiencies, etc.)

In all cases of a suspected disorder, children should be taken for diagnosis, because aside from postural problems, disorders in the lower extremities may also develop into motor gaps at a later age and impair overall functioning.

Regarding the lower extremities, special attention should be paid to the following:

- The foot (ankle joint balance and arch development)
- The knee joint (genu recurvatum, genu valgum/varum, tibial torsion)
- The hip joint – functional balance on the transverse plane in internal/external rotation movements.

(Detailed explanations of these disorders appear in Ch. 5.)

Postural characteristics of the feet in early childhood

The structure of the feet changes gradually as children grow. This is an important fact to take into account when diagnosing and treating children, because a child's age has a direct effect on how his or her feet function. In many cases, what is considered normal for a certain age is defined as a disorder at a later age (Gould & Davies, 1985).

In this context, one of the prominent characteristics of early childhood is low foot arches. This is normal for this age, since the arches continue to develop in later years. At the same time, children should be encouraged to exercise barefoot when possible and should have optimal conditions for foot growth (walking on toes, walking barefoot on sand, grass, carpets, mats, etc.). (Other examples for ways to strengthen foot arches are detailed in Ch. 8.)

Postural characteristics of the knee joints in early childhood

- Horizontal rotation of the tibia (tibial torsion) – in children, toeing-in may be the result of internal rotation of the tibia in relation to the femur (see also Ch. 5). Tibial torsion may also cause a toeing-out (depending on the rotational direction of the tibia) (Fig. 12.3). In these cases, it is important to obtain an orthopedic medical diagnosis, and on the basis of the data, to decide whether therapeutic intervention is warranted. In certain cases, joint positions may improve and even correct themselves spontaneously during the growth processes, and in other situations, medical intervention will be recommended.

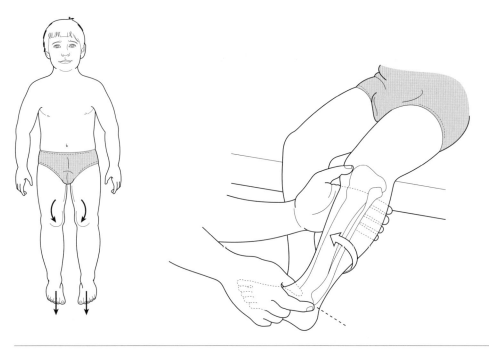

Figure 12.3 Tibial torsion in relation to the femur.

- Genu valgum/genu varum – in early childhood, a number of structural characteristics of the skeletal system affect lower extremity posture. Characteristic postural patterns are reflected in genu varum (bowlegs), which in most cases will improve spontaneously as children continue to develop (Kahle et al., 1986).

(Detailed explanation of these issues appears in Ch. 5, Figs 5.7 and 5.8.)

Postural characteristics of the hip joints in early childhood

Several disorders may develop in the hip joint because of a functional imbalance on the horizontal plane in internal–external rotation. Limited range of motion in internal or external hip rotation may cause an imbalance in walking and running, and impair children's motor functioning (faulty balance, a tendency to fall often, etc.). Aside from the motor implications, disorders of this kind also affect normal anatomical development of the hip joints (Norkin & Levangie, 1993).

Special attention should be paid to children's sitting habits. One of the common forms of children's sitting is a "W" position (Fig. 12.4). Although children may find this type of sitting comfortable and pleasant, it is not kinesiologically recommended, for the following reasons:

- The position overloads the medial aspect of the knee joints and may weaken the knee ligaments and undermine joint stability

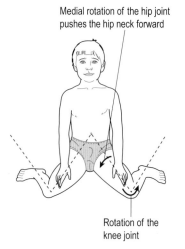

Medial rotation of the hip joint pushes the hip neck forward

Rotation of the knee joint

Figure 12.4 "W" sitting position.

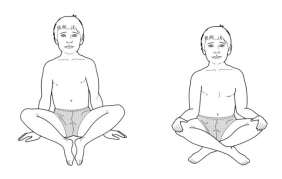

Figure 12.5 Sitting positions that create external hip rotation.

- Because the torsion angle of the femur tends to be greater in early childhood, this sitting position encourages a pushing forward of the femoral neck and although comfortable to the child, it prevents natural spontaneous correction (this is explained in greater detail later in this chapter).

This sitting position is especially problematic in conditions of excessive internal hip rotation, as it perpetuates and perhaps exacerbates the problem. Therefore, it is recommended to encourage children to sit in the cross-legged position or with their feet facing each other (Fig. 12.5).

This important change in movement and postural habits may have a positive effect on the normal development of the hip joints as the child undergoes natural growth processes.

When babies remain in a static position for extended periods of time, they can be gently shifted as they sleep. For those children with excessive internal or external rotation of the legs, it is possible to place their legs in proper balance during sleep. Support pillows can be used as needed to prevent legs from moving in an undesirable direction (Fig. 12.6).

Any change affecting young children's posture and physical development (including the use of any of the exercises or ideas in this chapter) should be carried out only under the guidance of an orthopedist and after professional diagnosis.

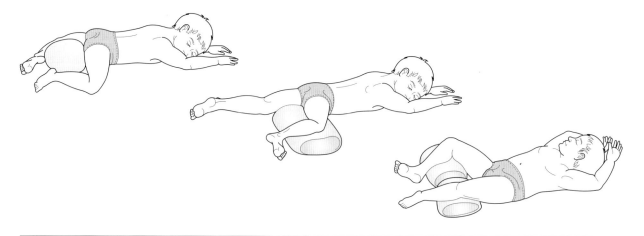

Figure 12.6 The use of support pillows to balance leg position during sleep.

Rotation movement mechanisms of the hip joint

One possible cause of excessive internal or external hip rotation is the anatomical position of the femoral neck in one of these two conditions:

- Anteversion
- Retroversion.

Under normal conditions (Fig. 12.7), the neck of the femur creates a 12° angle to the line connecting the two femoral condyles. This is the torsion angle of the femur (see also Ch. 5, Fig. 5.10). Any increase in this angle creates a condition called anteversion, which entails excessive internal rotation (Fig. 12.8). Such a condition may cause children to toe-in when they walk.

The reverse situation of anteversion is retroversion, where the torsion angle is <12°. Functionally, the result is excessive external rotation. While walking, the feet toe-out, much like Charlie Chaplin in his movies (Fig. 12.9).

In comparison to adults, young children are usually characterized by heightened anteversion torsion angle. This may explain the high prevalence of toddlers walking with their toes facing in (toe-in).

Summary

Physical maturity and correct instruction by kindergarten teachers, parents or school teachers may help ensure children's optimal development. An awareness of what constitutes optimal movement and postural development helps to prevent disorders from developing, and to treat them early if they appear.

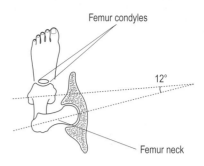
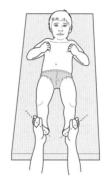
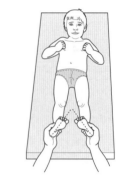

Figure 12.7 Normal anatomical position of the lower extremity joints.

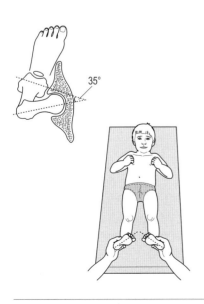

Figure 12.8 Anteversion position of the hip joint.

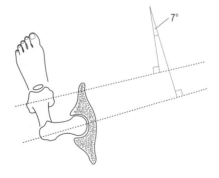

For measurement, vertical lines were drawn and the meeting point between them marks the torsion angle

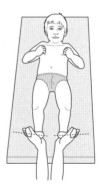

Figure 12.9 Retroversion position of the hip joint.

CHAPTER 13

Orthopedic support braces for treating children with postural disorders

After their initial attempts to obtain a reliable diagnosis and determine the appropriate treatment for their children, many parents feel frustrated by the often manifest differences between the opinions expressed by doctors and therapists.

In diagnosing a child with any kind of physical disability, professionals usually express little or no disagreement about the findings. But in cases of postural disorders, diagnoses can often be contradictory. The reason for these discrepancies lies in the substantial differences in the criteria each professional discipline employs. Thus, a child with minor symptoms of a postural disorder may be diagnosed in one of the following ways:

Option A: Because the disorder is minor, with no pains and no functional limitations, no treatment is recommended. The condition should simply be monitored periodically.

Option B: The child's problem may be diagnosed from other aspects, and even if no serious disorder is identified, treatment may be prescribed to prevent deterioration in the future, during the child's physical development (prescriptions include working on body awareness, changing movement and postural habits, and adapted exercise).

Option C: There is no need for specific movement treatment but swimming is recommended.

Extreme situations may occur in which an orthopedist may recommend the use of a brace of some type to treat a given child's minor postural problem, while another physician may totally dismiss any thought of treatment intervention.

In short, the diagnosis, interpretation of findings and recommendations offered depend on the professionals' subjective approach and their awareness of the side-effects of postural disorders (even if the disorders themselves do not entail serious pathologies).

This problem is often the cause of frustration and helplessness among parents as they deliberate on which approach to adopt. The only way to deal with such a situation is to use one's common sense and seek both the opinion of a medical expert and comprehensive diagnosis by a certified therapist with a movement orientation.

Each case *must* be examined on its own merits. In cases of severe disorders, the option of braces and other support apparatus should not be dismissed, but all cases in which braces are employed should also include adapted physical activity, which may enhance the effectiveness of the orthopedic treatment and reduce the chances of secondary damage caused by the apparatus (muscle weakness, movement rigidity, and affective damage).

Orthopedic support braces in therapy

The principle underlying treatment with orthopedic braces is the creation of mechanical supports that exert pressure on several points on the torso and spinal column. These supports are adapted specifically to the disorders and to the patient's physique (Kisner & Colby, 1985).

The main purposes of using a brace are to prevent further deterioration of a disorder in the spinal column and to provide general support and stability (mainly during the rapid growth spurt). The disorders in which support braces are used most commonly are idiopathic scoliosis (see Ch. 4), or severe cases of excessive curvatures on the sagittal plane, such as kyphosis or lordosis (see Ch. 3).

Of the various braces available, three are employed most often for treating severe postural disorders – the Milwaukee Brace, the Charleston Brace, and the Boston Brace. Variations on these braces, offering altered brace structure or different material composition, have been developed. The following are the main characteristics of each brace.

The Milwaukee Brace

The Milwaukee Brace (Fig. 13.1A,B) is used for orthopedic treatment of idiopathic scoliosis (see Ch. 4) in severe cases in which there is a fear of deterioration during the rapid growth spurt of adolescence. For this reason, the brace is not usually prescribed for adolescents who are past their growth spurt. At the same time, the brace may be prescribed for children under 10 years in whom severe scoliosis has been diagnosed.

The brace follows the direction of the scoliosis and is attached to the body. It creates support at several points along the spinal column in order to prevent the scoliosis from intensifying and to reduce rotation in the thoracic vertebrae.

The Milwaukee Brace is designed to allow "dynamic correction" of scoliosis in two ways:

1. The brace facilitates correction by providing mechanical supports that make children maintain better posture.
2. Use of the brace also encourages the integration of therapeutic exercise on a daily basis. The exercises are done with and without the brace.

In many cases, patients use the brace for 23 h/day, but exactly how many hours depends on parameters such as disorder severity, child's age and the attending orthopedist's approach. The results of studies investigating brace effectiveness and the number of hours per day it should be worn have varied widely (Donaldson, 1981).

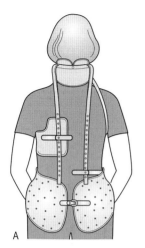

A

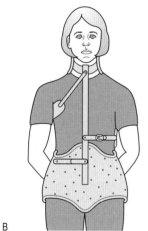

B

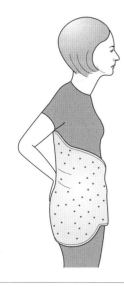

C

Figure 13.1 (A,B) The Milwaukee Brace and (C) the Charleston Brace.

Treatment effectiveness using the Milwaukee Brace is controversial, and the results depend on a variety of factors. Certain cases show significant improvement, while others manifest progressively worsening conditions of scoliosis despite the brace. Even when spinal alignment has improved, it is possible that once the brace is removed the condition may gradually regress to its previous state.

These findings are frustrating because the treatment results are not always clear. At the same time, the risk exists that not using the brace will allow the disorder to deteriorate even more. Therefore, it is recommended to weigh all the factors, obtain a number of opinions, and not dismiss the use of the brace out of hand only because of its discomfort.

The Charleston Brace

The Charleston Brace (Fig. 13.1C) was developed for the same conditions as the Milwaukee Brace but is more comfortable for children to use. In many cases, the brace is worn only at night when the child is sleeping.

The Boston Brace

The Boston Brace is used mainly for supporting the torso and does not affect the cervical spine. This brace is most commonly used in case of serious postural disorders in the sagittal plane such as rounded back, kyphosis or lordosis, but in certain cases it is an effective means of support for scoliosis as well.

Main aspects in the use of orthopedic braces

As noted, the use of braces is still controversial, and it is recommended that the decision be made after weighing both the drawbacks and the benefits of such treatment. A later section of this chapter will provide recommendations about when the use of a brace is indicated.

Advantages of using a support brace

- The brace may provide vital stability for the spinal column. In cases of severe disorders, the brace can help to prevent the condition from deteriorating during the growth spurt by means of mechanical support that prevents the spinal column from collapsing in the direction of the deviation
- The brace may help to improve ranges of motion limited by shortened muscles, by means of prolonged mechanical pressure from the brace that may with time stretch the short muscles. In many cases of kyphosis accompanied by a shortening of the pectoral muscles and a pulling forward of the shoulders, the Boston Brace may be helpful and prevent the shoulders from being pulled forward into scapular protraction (Fig. 13.2).

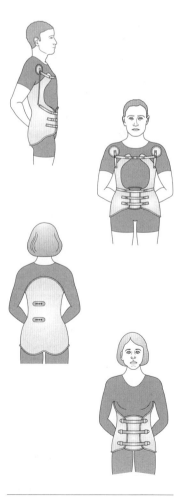

Figure 13.2 The Boston Brace.

Disadvantages of support braces

- An uncomfortable period of adjustment. Usually this feeling decreases with time
- Changes in movement patterns caused by significant restrictions on range of torso motion, which affects movement control and the quality of children's motor performance. Conspicuous examples are new walking patterns children devise as well as new ways of writing and performing other daily functions, such as dressing and eating
- Limitation of respiratory functioning as a result of pressure on the chest. This pressure may restrict inhalation volume and create shallow, short breathing
- The brace must be adjusted every few months because of the children's process of growth
- Prolonged use of support braces may create points of pressure in other parts of the body and limit range of motion. This will be reflected in rigid movement patterns and a sensitivity to injury and pains
- Because the brace creates mechanical support, it may weaken postural muscles by subsuming their function of stabilizing the torso
- Use of the brace may affect the child's self esteem and social functioning. This depends to a great extent on the child's personality and social status.

When using a brace it is important to remember:

- Lying down (on one's back) several times a day may give a feeling of relief and rest
- Sleeping on a not-overly-firm mattress may ease discomfort (in cases where a child is supposed to sleep with the brace)
- It is advisable to adapt clothing to the brace and use wide, lightweight clothing
- It is advisable to learn and practice breathing exercises to increase ranges of inhalation and exhalation (see Ch. 8). These exercises should be performed without the brace, while lying on the back, making maximal use of chest and rib movement
- Together with the breathing exercises, it is advisable to perform special exercises for pelvic position, tilting it forward and backward. Such exercise is also important for strengthening the abdominal muscles.

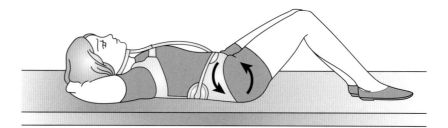

Figure 13.3 Anterior and posterior pelvic tilt as can be done with or without the brace.

The importance of combining brace support treatment with adapted physical activity

Physical activity is an important element of treatment whenever a brace is utilized. Some of the exercises can be performed without the brace and others with the brace on (Fig. 13.3). The main aims of therapeutic exercise in these cases are:

- Maintaining muscle strength throughout the torso because activity declines significantly as a result of the fixating support of the brace. This maintenance is especially important for optimal functioning when brace treatment ceases
- Maintaining normal ranges of motion, which is important for the spinal areas fixated as a result of the brace and also for other areas such as the shoulder girdle and the hip joints
- Working on cardiopulmonary endurance by means of activity not entailing shocks and vertical loads on the spine, such as work on stationary bicycles, swimming, etc.
- Improving functional balance between antagonist muscle groups in the torso and along the spinal column. When necessary, asymmetrical exercises especially adapted to the patient's specific disorder and symptoms should be performed
- General sport activity according to what the children like (swimming, ball games, etc.). Except for activities that are contraindicated (depending on the problem), it is recommended that children be encouraged to participate in sports activities, which may contribute to their physical, social, and emotional well-being. It is important to remember that movement games and sports serve as important channels of communications for children, and every effort should be made to avoid social isolation caused by abstention from physical activity. Physical activity has many important ramifications for the self esteem and physical image that children develop about themselves.

Summary

The effectiveness of treatment with braces and other devices is contro-versial. The approach recommended in this chapter is not extreme in either direction – it does not reject the use of any device outright, nor does it unequivocally advocate its use.

Each case must be examined on its own merits and the decision should be made on the basis of a comprehensive diagnosis that takes the following parameters into account:

- The severity of the disorder
- The child's emotional state
- Concern about possible worsening of the disorder without use of a brace
- Concern about possible damage as a result of using the brace (emotional problems, damage to self esteem, avoidance of physical activity, weakening of muscles, etc.).

CHAPTER 14

Methodological aspects in the treatment of children with postural disorders

This chapter will discuss a number of methodo–
logical aspects of instruction and treatment in
dealing with postural disorders. Therapists who
understand and implement these aspects will be
better equipped to plan their work and choose the
most appropriate materials and teaching methods
for their patients without clinging to unchanging,
rigid exercise patterns.

Aims of treatment in postural disorders

Normal posture, which provides a foundation for optimal body movement, is intrinsically intertwined, as mentioned, with various aspects of human anatomy and physiology. Mechanically speaking, body joints and bones should be aligned for the most efficient bearing of loads resulting from body movement and body weight.

Balanced posture is almost impossible without balance between antagonist muscle groups. Problems there may cause an imbalance in skeletal alignment and over-load joints in the lower extremities, the pelvis or the spine. Therapists must accurately pinpoint the main factors producing the postural disorder and basing themselves on this initial diagnosis, determine the aims of the treatment.

Main treatment aims in postural disorders deal with the following:

- Maintaining joint mobility and improving functional balance between antagonist muscle groups in order to correct postural disorders on the various planes (such as kyphosis, scoliosis, lordosis, etc.)
- Improving specific motor functions that particularly affect posture or are affected by it, such as balance and coordination. One of the aims of treatment is to create the conditions for "natural" body functioning by means of a balanced distribution of energy, where each part of the system functions in coordination with the other parts. This is the actual meaning of normal posture patterns
- Creating and preserving a new body image – altering wrong habits of movement and posture and learning correct ones. Just as a plant needs water for its roots, not its leaves, mechanically performing one "exercise" or another is not enough. To bring about true change, patients must locate the source of their problem and create change at that specific point.

Individuals exposed to lessons that integrate therapeutic exercise, experience a variety of movement options that allows them to broaden their movement options and better understand how body limbs interact functionally.

It is extremely important to include postural exercises that help to improve body image. These should include relaxation exercises for reducing excess muscle tone, static and dynamic balance exercises, exercises to improve respiratory functioning, and exercises to develop kinesthetic sense in movement with eyes open and closed.

Selecting the treatment design

Treatment of postural disorders can be given individually or in groups. Each format has its benefits. After the diagnostic stage, therapists should select the optimal treatment by considering the type and severity of the disorder, the child's personality and the working conditions, such as the type and size of the facility available.

The recommended therapeutic approach usually strives to have children progress and become integrated in group activities. At the same time, coping with significant postural disorders often requires a preliminary period of individual activities.

The individual treatment format has a number of advantages

- Better adaptation of the treatment program to the child's needs. Individualized treatment allows the therapist to become more familiar with the child's inner world. In this format, therapists can talk with the child, be attentive to his or her special desires and learn about weaknesses and about those things he or she "loves" or "hates".

  On the physical–postural plane, such familiarity with the child makes adaptation of the exercises to specific problems more accurate. This is especially important in disorders entailing special asymmetric exercise, such as in treating scoliosis (see Ch. 9, Fig. 9.23)
- The possibility of incorporating treatment techniques involving touch, including methods for strengthening and relaxing muscles, and manipulations that allow passive mobilization of the various joints
- Better monitoring of performance quality of postural exercises the children learn during the treatment
- Easier and better monitoring of children's progress through periodic tests that check the treatment effect on the disorder.

Stages of individual treatment for children with postural disorders

Individual treatment may include a number of stages, as illustrated in Figure 14.1. For children to derive maximum pleasure and benefit from therapeutic activity, and to maintain a high level of motivation over time, each therapeutic meeting should include three components:

1. The learning component – children learn and gradually internalize what is being taught.
2. The pleasure and game component – movement games and psychomotor tasks adapted to the problem under treatment (see Ch. 11, Fig. 11.1 for an example).
3. The therapeutic component – specific attention to the patient's special needs. Here, in addition to specific exercises, therapists can employ the special tools at their disposal, such as flexibility techniques and touch therapies (massages, passive mobilization, resistance exercises, etc.) (see Ch. 9).

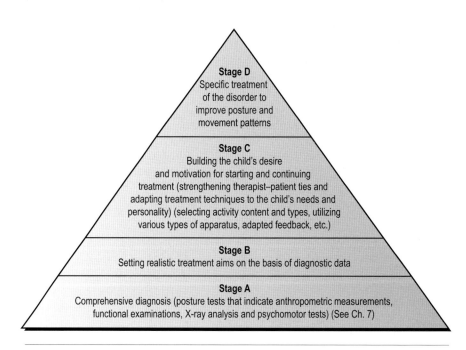

Figure 14.1 Stages of individual treatment for children with postural disorders.

Afterword

In contrast to disciplines with clearly defined and acknowledged boundaries such as physical therapy or occupational therapy, it is hard to find one term that encompasses the entire range of interventions detailed in this book. Movement and postural patterns, both in terms of learning processes and of functional aspects, cannot be defined exclusively as the function of physiological processes in the musculoskeletal system. Despite the considerable influence of various emotional processes on human movement, many of the ties that link parallel neurophysiological and psychological processes are missing. The approach presented in this book emphasizes the integrative nature of many of the components (some of them anatomical–physiological, others behavioral–affective) that affect movement and postural traits. It is little wonder, then, that such an integrative approach is quite naturally applied to a field that focuses on adapted physical activity for populations with special needs.

The material presented in this book is based on generally accepted principles in motor development, kinesiology, and biomechanics, but the many ideas and exercises presented here are applied illustrations that therapists are invited to alter, expand on, and deepen. Like any good plan, this book should serve as a basis for change. This approach strives to employ the principles described as the basis for developing additional therapeutic tools. Each exercise presented here can be developed into a more comprehensive movement process, and each motor task cited as an example can be adapted and adjusted to an individual patient's special needs.

In other words, the spirit of this book encourages the use of what has been done as a basis for developing new ideas and materials: "creating" instead of "buying", "exporting" instead of "importing". In this way, we will mutually enrich one another with fascinating materials and a therapeutic approach that encourages flexibility and variety in thought. Chapter 6, which deals with diagnostic approaches, mentions "Maslov's hammer". It is my hope that this book will contribute another tool or two to each reader's personal tool chest.

References

Adams, J. A. (1971) A closed-loop theory of motor learning. Journal of Motor Behavior, 3, 111–149.

Alter, M. J. (1988) Science of Stretching, 1st edn. Illinois: BA Brooks.

Arroyo, J. S., Hershon, S. J. & Bigliani, L. U. (1997) Special considerations in the athletic throwing shoulder. Orthopedic Clinics of North America, 28(1), 69–77.

Baharav, A. (1972) Sport Injuries. Tel Aviv: Niv.

Bak, K. (1996) Nontraumatic glenohumeral instability and coracoacromial impingement in swimmers. Scandinavian Journal of Medicine & Science in Sports, 6, 132–144.

Bak, K. and Faunl, P. (1997) Clinical findings in competitive swimmers with shoulder pain. The American Journal of Sports Medicine, 25(2), 254–260.

Basmajian, J. V. & Slonecker, C. E. (1989) Method of Anatomy: A Clinical Problem Solving Approach, 11th edn. Baltimore: Williams & Wilkins.

Basmajian, J. V. (1978) Therapeutic Exercise, 3rd edn. Baltimore: Williams & Wilkins.

Bergman, A. & Hutzler, Y. (1996) Rehabilitation in Water. Ramat Gan: Alef Alef Press.

Brown, L. (1988) An introduction to the treatment and examination of the spine by combined movements. Journal of the Chartered Society of Physiotherapists, 74(7), 347–353.

Buscaglia, L. (1982) Living, Loving and Learning. Tel Aviv: Zamora.

Chia, M. (1993) Iron Shirt Chi Kung. New York: Healing Tao Books.

Chukuka, S., Enwemeka, I., Bonet, M. I., Jayanti, A. I., Prudhithomrong, S. & Ogbahon, E. F. (1986) Postural correction in persons with neck pain. Journal of Orthopaedic and Sports Physical Therapy, 8(5), 235–238.

Cyriax, J. (1979) Textbook of Orthopaedic Medicine, 7th edn. London: Baillière Tindall and Cassell.

Dennis, M. (1976) Impaired sensory and motor differentiation with corpus callosum agenesis: a lack of callosal inhibition during ontogeny. Neuropsychologia, 14(4), 456–469.

Donaldson, W. F. (1981) Scoliosis. In: A.B. Ferguson, ed. Orthopedic Surgery in Infancy and Childhood, 5th edn. Baltimore: Williams and Wilkins.

Enoka R. M. (1994) Neuromechanical Basis of Kinesiology, 2nd edn. Champaign, IL: Human Kinetics.

Fuchs, Z., Ben-Sira, D. & Zaichkovsky, L. (1985) Selected Issues in Motor Learning, Part 2: Psycho-neurological and Developmental Aspects. Netanya: Wingate Institute, Gil Publishers.

Geissele, M. E., Kransdorf, M. J., Geyer, C. A., Jelinwk, J. S. & Van Dam, B. E. (1991) Idiopathic scoliosis and asymmetry of form and function. Spine, 16(7): 761–763.

Glousman, R. (1993) Electromyographic analysis and its role in the athletic shoulder. Clinical Orthopaedics and Related Research, 288, 27–34.

Gould, J. A. & Davies, G. J. (1985) Orthopaedic and Sports Physical Therapy, Vol. 2. Princeton: C.V. Mosby.

Gur, V. (1998a) The Posture Cultivation Department – Handbook for third and fourth year students in the department. The Zinman College of Physical Education and Sport Sciences at the Wingate Institute.

Gur, V. (1998b). Muscle stretches: The anatomy and biomechanics of connective tissues. Physical Education and Sport, 7, 5–9.

Gur, V. (1998c) The neurophysiology of muscle stretching – Theoretical background and accepted techniques. Physical Education and Sport, 2, 11–16.

Gur, V. (1999a) Issues in flexibility. Physical Education and Sport, 3, 10–14.

Gur, V. (1999b) The hamstrings: characteristics and methods of lengthening them. Physical Education and Sport, 6, 8–14.

Hales, T. R. & Bernard, B. P. (1996) Epidemiology of work related musculoskeletal disorders. Orthopedic Clinics of North America, 27, 679–709.

Hamilton, N. & Luttgens, K. (2002) Kinesiology: Scientific Basis of Human Motion, 10th edn. New York, NY: McGraw-Hill.

Heijden, G., Beurskens, A., Dirx, M., Bouter, L. M. & Lindeman, E. (1995) Efficacy of lumbar traction: A randomized clinical trial. Physiotherapy, 81, 29–35.

Hess, S. A. (2000) Functional stability of the glenohumeral joint. Manual Therapy, 5(2), 63–71.

Holon Center for Therapeutic Sport (2000) A Diagnostic Model: Exercises for Evaluating a Child's Functional Ability in Therapeutic Sport. Holon: Solberg.

Hoppenfeld, S. (1976) Physical Examination of the Spine and Extremities. New York, NY: Prentice Hall.

Hutzler, Y. (1990) Psychomotorics in education and rehabilitation. Physical Education and Sport, 6, 5–7.

Kahle, W., Leonhardt, H. & Platzer, W. (1986) Locomotor System, Color Atlas/Text of Human Anatomy, Vol. 1. New York: Thieme Verlag.

Kamkar, A., Irrgang, J. J. & Whitney, S. L. (1993) Nonoperative management of secondary shoulder impingement syndrome. Journal of Orthopaedic and Sports Physical Therapy, 17(5), 212–224.

Keim, H. R. (1982) The Adolescent Spine, 1st edn. New York: Springer Verlag.

Kendall, F. & McCreary, E. K. (1983) Muscles: testing and function, 3rd edn. Baltimore: Williams and Wilkins.

Kephart, N. C. (1960) The Slow Learner in the Classroom. Columbus, OH: Merrill.

Kibler, W. B. (1998) The role of the scapula in athletic shoulder function. American Journal of Sports Medicine, 26(2), 325–337.

Kibler, W. B., Uhl, T. L. & Maddux, J. W. (2002) Qualitative clinical evaluation of scapular dysfunction: a reliability study. Journal of Shoulder and Elbow Surgery, 11(6), 550–556.

Kisner, C. & Colby, L. A. (1985) Therapeutic Exercise, 2nd edn. Philadelphia: F. A. Davis.

Lippitt, S. & Matsen, F. (1993) Mechanisms of glenohumeral joint stability. Clinical Orthopaedics and Related Research, 291, 20–28.

Loncar-Dusek, M., Pecina, M. & Preberg, Z. (1991) A longitudinal study of growth velocity and development of secondary gender characteristics versus onset of idiopathic scoliosis. Clinical Orthopaedics and Related Research, 270(1), 278–282.

Ludewig, P. M. & Cook, T. M. (2000) Alterations in shoulder kinematics and associated muscle activity in people with symptoms of shoulder impingement. Physical Therapy, 80(3), 276–291.

McQuade, K. J., Dawson, J. & Smidt, G. L. (1998). Scapulothoracic muscle fatigue associated with alterations in scapulohumeral rhythm kinematics during maximum resistive shoulder elevation. Journal of Orthopaedic and Sports Physical Therapy, 28(2), 74–80.

Mitrany, R. (1993) Sport Injuries: Diagnosis, Treatment and Prevention of Physical Injuries as a Result of Athletic Activity. Netanya: Wingate Institute, Gil Publishers.

Nachemson, A. (1983) The load on the lumbar disks in different positions of the body. Clinics in Orthopedics, 45, 107–122.

Nicolopoulus, K. S., Burwell, R. G. & Webb, J. K. (1985) Stature and its component in adolescent idiopathic scoliosis: Cephalo-caudal disproportion in the trunk of girls. Journal of Bone and Joint Surgery, 67(13), 594–601.

Nordin, M. & Frankel, V. H. (1989) Basic Biomechanics of the Musculoskeletal System, 2nd edn. Philadelphia: Lea & Febiger.

Norkin, C. & Levangie, P. (1993) Joint Structure and Function: A Comprehensive Analysis. Philadelphia: F. A. Davis.

Nudelman, W. & Reis, N. D. (1990) Anatomy of the extrinsic spinal muscles related to the deformity of scoliosis. Acta Anatomica, 139(3), 220–225.

Nudelman, W. & Reis, N. D. (1990) Anatomy of the extrinsic spinal muscles related to the deformity of scoliosis. Acta Anatomica, 139(3), 220–225.

Rasch, P. S. (1989) Kinesiology and Applied Anatomy, 7th edn. Philadelphia: Lea & Febiger.

Ratzon, M. (1993) Perceptual Motor Development and Learning Processes. Tel Aviv: Seminar Hakibbutzim Press.

Ratzon, M. (1993) Perceptual Motor Development and Learning Processes. Tel Aviv: Seminar Hakibbutzim Press.

Ratzon, M. (1993). Perceptual Motor Development and Learning Processes. Tel Aviv: Seminar Hakibbutzim Press.

Roaf, R. (1978) Posture, 1st edn. London: Academic Press.

Sandor, R. & Brone, S. (2000) Exercising the frozen shoulder. Physician and Sportsmedicine, 28(9), 83–84.

Schmidt, R.A. (1988) Motor Control and Learning: A Behavioral Emphasis. Champaign, IL: Human Kinetics.

Schmitt, L. & Snyder-Mackler, L. (1999) The role of scapular stabilizers in etiology and treatment of impingement syndrome. Journal of Orthopaedic and Sports Physical Therapy, 29(1), 31–38.

Schroth, C. (1992). Introduction to the three dimensional scoliosis treatment according to Schroth. Physiotherapy, 78(11), 810–815.

Sherington, C. S. (1906) The Integrative Action of the Nervous System. Cambridge: Saunders.

Snir, D. (1996) Medical aspects of hydrotherapy. In: A. Bergman & Y. Hutzler, eds., Rehabilitation in Water. Ramat Gan: Alef Alef Press.

Solberg, G. (1994) Diagnosing scoliosis. Physical Education and Sport, 1, 5–7.

Solberg, G. (1995) Activity in the water as therapy for postural disorders. Physical Education and Sport, 5, 11–14.

Solberg, G. (1996a). Plastic changes in spinal function of pre-pubescent scoliotic children engaged in an exercise therapy program. South African Journal of Physiotherapy, 52(1), 19–22.

Solberg, G. (1996b) Posture Cultivation and Therapeutic Exercise: Handbook for Teachers and Therapists. Tel Aviv: Solberg.

Solberg, G. (1998a) Comprehensive psychomotor diagnosis for populations with special needs (Part I). Physical Education and Sport, 1, 10–13.

Solberg, G. (1998b) Comprehensive psychomotor diagnosis for populations with special needs (Part II). Physical Education and Sport, 2, 25–28.

Solberg, G. (1999) Comprehensive psychomotor diagnosis for populations with special needs (Part III). Physical Education and Sport, 3, 32–34.

Spirduso, W. W. (1978) Hemispheric lateralization and orientation in compensatory and voluntary movement, In: G. E. Stelmach, ed. Information Processing in Motor Control and Learning. New York: Academic Press.

Steindler, A. (1970) Kinesiology of the Human Body Under Normal and Pathological Conditions, 2nd edn. Springfield: Charles C. Thomas.

Stokes, I. A. & Gardner, M. M. (1991) Analysis of the interaction between vertebral lateral deviation and axial rotation in scoliosis. Journal of Biomechanics, 24(8), 753–759.

Stone, B., Beekman, C., Hall, V., Guess, V. & Brooks, L. (1979) The effect of an exercise program on change in curve in adolescents with minimal idiopathic scoliosis, Physical Therapy, 59(6), 759–763.

Swarts, L. (1978) Role of kinaesthesia in arousal and learning behavior. Perceptual and Motor Skills, 47, 1219–1225.

Taylor, D. C. & Arciero, R. A. (1997) Pathologic changes associated with shoulder dislocations: arthroscopic and physical examination findings in first-time, traumatic anterior dislocations. American Journal of Sports Medicine, 25(3), 306–311.

Taylor, J. R. (1983). Scoliosis and growth: Patterns of asymmetry in normal vertebral growth. Acta Orthopaedica Scandinavica, 54(1), 596–602.

Thein, L. A. & Greenfield, B. H. (1997) Impingement syndrome and impingement-related instability. In R. A. Donatelli, ed. Physical Therapy of the Shoulder, 3rd edn., pp. 240–254. New York: Churchill Livingstone.

Tyler, T. F., Nicholas, S. J. & Roy, T. (2000) Quantification of posterior capsule tightness and motion loss in patients with shoulder impingement. American Journal of Sports Medicine, 28(5), 668–673.

Waddell, G. (1996) Low back pain: A twentieth century health care enigma. Spine, 21, 2820–2825.

Wagner, H. (1990). Pelvis tilt and leg length correction. Orthopedische, 19(5), 273–277.

Warner, J. J., Micheli L. J. & Arslanian, L. E. (1990) Patterns of flexibility, laxity and strength in normal shoulders and shoulders with instability and impingement. American Journal of Sports Medicine, 18(4), 366–375.

Warner, J., Micheli, L. J. & Arslanian, L. E. (1992) Scapulothoracic motion in normal shoulders and shoulders with glenohumeral instability and impingement syndrome: a study using Moire topographic analysis. Clinical Orthopaedics, 285, 191–199.

White, S. & Carmeli, A. (1999) Shoulder pains in swimmers. Physical Education and Sport, 5.

Wilk, K. E., Meister K., Andrews, J. R. (2002) Current concepts in the rehabilitation of the overhead throwing athlete. American Journal of Sports Medicine, 30(1), 136–151.

Yakovlev, P. I. & Lencours, A. R. (1967) The myelogenetics cycles of regional maturation of the brain. In: A. Minkowsky, ed. Regional Development of the Brain in Early Life. Oxford: Blackwell.

Yazdi-Ugav, O. (1995) Motor Development and Motor Learning – Normal vs Abnormal: Theoretical and Practical Aspects. Netanya, Israel: Wingate Institute, Emmanuel Gill Publishing.

Bibliography

Amendt, L. E., Ause Ellias, K. L., Eybers, J. L., Wadsworth, C. T., Nielsen, D. H. & Weinstein, S. L. (1990) Validity and reliability of the scoliometer. Physical Therapy, 70, 108–117.

Anderson, G. B. & Deyo, R. A. (1996) History and examination in patients with herniated discs. Spine, 21, 10–18.

Arad, H. (1993) Work Program for Physical Education Teachers in Special Education. Netanya: Wingate Institute, Gil Publishers.

Aikin, A. M. (1950) The mechanism of rotation in combination with lateral deviation in the normal spine. Journal of Bone and Joint Surgery, 32(A), 180–190.

Astrand, P. (1992) Why exercise? Medicine and Science in Sports and Exercise, 24, 153–162.

Auxter, D., Pyfer, J. & Huettig, C. (1997) Principles and Methods of Adapted Physical Education and Recreation, 8th edn. St Louis, MO: Mosby-Year Book.

Axelgard, J. & Brown, J. C. (1983) Lateral electrical surface stimulation for the treatment of progressive idiopathic scoliosis. Spine, 8, 242–260.

Bachara, G. H. (1976) Empathy in learning disabled children. Perceptual and Motor Skills, 43, 541–542.

Barlow, W. (1975) The Alexander Principle. London: Arrow Books.

Basmajian, J. V. (1985) Manipulation, Traction, and Massage, 3rd edn. Baltimore: Williams & Wilkins.

Bergman, A. (1996) Swimming for Populations with Special Needs: A Resource Book for Students, Teachers and Coaches. Tel Aviv: Seminar Hakibbutzim Teachers' College.

Bohannon, R. (1985) Contribution of pelvic and lower limb motion to increase in the angle of passive straight leg raising. Physical Therapy, 65, 4, 474–476.

Broer, M. & Zernicke, R (1979) Efficiency of Human Movement, 5th edn. Philadelphia: Saunders Company.

Bunnell, W. P. (1984) An objective criterion for scoliosis screening. Journal of Bone and Joint Surgery, 66, 1381–1387.

Calais-Germain, B. (1993) Anatomy of Movement. Seattle: Eastland Press.

Capasso, G., Maffulli, N. & Testa, V. (1992) The validity and reliability of measurements in spinal deformities: a critical appraisal. Acta Orthopaedica Belgica, 58(2), 126–135.

Connor-Kuntz, F. J., Dummer, G. M. & Paciorek, M. J. (1995) Physical education and sport participation of children and youth with Spina Bifida Myelomeningocele. Adapted Physical Activity Quarterly, 12, 228–238.

Cornbleet, S. (1966) Assessment of hamstrings muscle length in school children. Physical Therapy, 76, 8, 850–855.

Daniels, L. & Worthingham, C. (1980) Muscle Testing: Techniques of Manual Examination. Philadelphia: W.B. Saunders.

Davis, W. E. & Rizzo, T. (1991) Issues in the classification of motor disorders. Adapted Physical Activity Quarterly, 8, 280–304.

Donatell, R. (1987) Abnormal biomechanics of the foot and ankle. Journal of Orthopaedic Sports and Physical Therapy, 9, 11–16.

Dun, John M. (1989) Special Physical Education: Adapted, Individualized, Developmental, 6th edn. Dubuque, Iowa: W.C. Brown.

Farfan, H. (1995) Musculoskeletal system as revealed by mathematical analysis of the lumbar spine. Spine, 20, 1462–1474.

Gajdosik, R. (1992) Influence of short hamstrings muscles on the pelvis and lumbar spine in standing and during the toe-touch test. Clinical Biomechanics, 7, 38–42.

Giallonardo, L. (1988) Clinical evaluation of foot and ankle dysfunction. Physical Therapy, 68, 1850–1856.

Gur, V. (1988) "Permitted" and "forbidden" flexibility exercises. Physical Education and Sport, 6, 8–14.

Hadler, N. M. (1995) Controversy. Low back school. Education or exercise? Spine, 20, 1098.

Halbertsma, J. & Goeken, L. (1996) Sport stretching: Effect on passive muscle stiffness of short hamstrings. Archives of Physical Medicine and Rehabilitation, 77, 688–692.

Hutzler, Y. (1995) Movement on Wheelchairs: A Guide for Users and Therapists. Haifa: Achva Publishers.

Hutzler, Y, Raz-Liberman, Z., Lidor, R. & Liberman, D. (1995) Control and Motor Learning in Physical Education and Sport: Fundamentals, Approaches and Implementation. Netanya: Wingate Institute, Gil Publishers.

Jansma, P. (1994) Special Physical Education: Physical Activity, Sports and Recreation. Englewood Cliffs, N.J.: Prentice Hall.

Kerrigan, C., Deming L. C. & Molden M. K. (1996) Knee recurvatum in gait: a study of associated knee biomechanics. Archives of Physical Medicine and Rehabilitation, 77, 645–650.

Kisner, C. & Colby, L. A. (1985) Therapeutic Exercise, 2nd edn. Philadelphia: F.A. Davis.

Koeslag, J. H. (1993) What is normal? South African Medical Journal, 83(1), 47–50.

Krau, G. (1981) Problems with Children – Signs and Symptoms of Difficulties in Early Childhood. Tel Aviv: Reshafim.

Li, Y. L. & McClure, P. (1996) The effect of hamstrings muscle stretching on standing posture and on lumbar and hip motions during forward bending. Physical Therapy, 76, 8, 836–849.

Manniche, C. & Hesselsoe, G. (1991) Intensive dynamic back exercises for chronic low back pain: a clinical trial. Pain, 47, 53–56.

McGill, S. (1998) Low back exercises: Evidence for improving exercise regimens. Physical Therapy, 78, 7, 755–764.

Muhugh, E. (1995) The role of aquatic programs in facilities serving children with physical disabilities. Clinical Kinesiology, 48(4), 83–84.

Osternig, L. R., Robertson R. N., Troxel R. K. & Hansen P. (1990) Differential responses to proprioceptive neuromuscular facilitation (PNF) stretch techniques. Medicine and Science in Sports and Exercise, 22(1), 106–111.

Prustig, M. (1994) Move, Grow, Learn: Movement Education – A Teacher's Guide and Set of New Updated Exercises. Tel Aviv: National Center for Special Education.

Reid, G. (1992) Editorial on theory, exchange and terminology. Adapted Physical Activity Quarterly, 9, 1–4.

Rolf, I. (1977) Structural Integration: The Re-Creation of the Balanced Human Body. New York, NY: Viking Press.

Rose, G., Welton, E. & Marshall, T. (1984) The diagnosis of flat foot in the child. Journal of Bone and Joint Surgery, 8, 71–78.

Russel, J. P. (1988) Graded Activities for Children with Motor Difficulties. Cambridge: Cambridge University Press.

Sacks, O. (1990) The Man Who Mistook His Wife for a Hat. Tel Aviv: Zamora.

Schwarzer, A. C., Aprill, C. N. & Bogduk, N. (1995) The sacroiliac joint in chronic low back pain. Spine, 20, 31–37.

Shahar-Levy, T. (1994) Initial memory aggregates: Mobility as a code of enciphering and revitalizing pre-cognitive memories. Conversations, 8 (3).

Sharan, S. & Sharan, Y. (1981) Learning Disorders and Their Remediation. Tel Aviv: Sifriat Hapoalim.

Sherill, C. (1993) Adapted Physical Activity, Recreation and Sport: Crossdisciplinary and Lifespan, 4th edn. Dubuque, IO: Brown and Benchmark.

Sherington, C. (1906) On the proprioceptive system, especially in its reflex aspect, Brain, 29, 467–482.

Sherman, A. (1995) Physical Education and Sport for Populations with Special Needs. Netanya: Wingate Institute, Gil Publishers.

Sherman, A. (1995) Physical Education for the Special Child. Netanya: Wingate Institute, Gil Publishing.

Simpson, S. & Baharav, Y. (1979) Diagnosing and Promoting the Special Child of Kindergarten Age. Tel Aviv: Ahiasaf.

Solberg, G. (1991) Posture cultivation and therapeutic exercise in the Holon Center for Therapeutic Sport. Physical Education and Sport, 1, 17–19.

Solberg, G. (1993) Is there a universal standard for good posture? Physical Education and Sport, 3, 18–19.

Solberg, G. (1994) The effect of therapeutic exercise on scoliosis. Physical Education and Sport, 2, 6–8.

Solberg, G. (1997) Belly-Back – Handbook for Combat Fitness Instructors. Netanya: Ministry of Defense.

Stokes, I. A. (1991) Biomechanical Testing and Scoliosis: In Vivo Methods. Spine, 16(10), 1217–1223.

Van Coppenolle, H., Simons, J., Pierloot, R. Probst, M. & Kanapen, J. (1989) The Louvain Observation scales for objectives in psychomotor therapy. Adapted Physical Activity Quarterly, 6(2), 170–175.

Warner, J. J. P. (1992) Scapulothoracic motion in normal shoulders and shoulders with glenohumeral instability and impingement syndrome. Clinical Orthopaedics and Related Research, 295, 191–199.

Wells, K. (1966) Kinesiology, 4th edn. Philadelphia: Saunders Company.

Williams, P. L. & Warwick, C. L. (1989) Gray's Anatomy, 37th edn. New York: Churchill Livingstone.

Wynarsky, G. T. & Shultz, A. B. (1991) Optimization of skeletal configuration: Studies of scoliosis correction biomechanics. Journal of Biomechanics, 24(8), 721–732.

Yalom, E. (1991) Love's Hangman. Tel Aviv: Kineret.

Appendix 1

Diagnostic intake report

Date: _____

First & Surname: _____ Gender: M / F (circle one)

Address: _____

Age: _____ Telephone (Home): _____ (Work): _____

Referred by: _____

General information

Pregnancy: _____

Birth: _____

General development: Senses (sight, hearing, touch sensitivity): _____
_____

Motor development (developmental stages) _____

Overall motor functioning _____

Diseases – Allergies _____

Pains _____

Medication _____

Physical activity _____

Club activity _____

Additional treatment _____

General information about the problem and its development _____
_____
_____
_____
_____
_____

Appendix 2

Parameters for emotional reference

Date: _____

Patient's name: _____

1. Organizing for and coping with a task _____
2. Social communication _____
3. Self confidence _____
4. Frustration threshold _____
5. Motivation _____
6. Impulsivity – Aggressiveness _____
7. Hyperactivity/hypoactivity _____
8. Emotional expression _____
9. Self esteem _____
10. Fears _____
_____
_____
_____
_____

Appendix 3

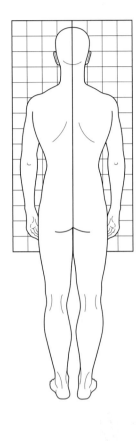

Posture examination form

Date: _____

Name: _____

Surname: _____

Gender: M / F

Date of birth: _____

General Examination

a. Posterior view

1. Achilles tendon and feet: Right _____ Left _____
2. Knees (genu varum/genu valgum) _____
3. Pelvic balance (posterior/superior iliac spine) _____
4. Scapulae (height, distance from spine, rotation) _____
5. Shoulder line _____
6. Neck _____
7. Symmetry of fat folds (pelvis, waist, neck) _____
8. Spinal column (scoliosis) _____

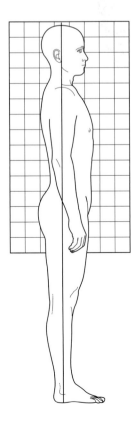

b. Lateral view

1. Feet arches _____
2. Knees (hyperextension) _____
3. Pelvis (posterior/anterior tilt) _____
4. Spinal curves (kyphosis/lordosis/flat back) _____
5. Shoulder position _____
6. Head position (cervical lordosis) _____

c. Anterior view

1. Feet _____
2. Knees _____
3. Pelvis (anterior superior iliac spine) _____
4. Shoulders height _____
5. Neck/Head _____

Functional tests (Figs 7.1–7.13)

1. Length of spinal column (C7–S1) _____
   Standing _____ Forward bending _____
2. General flexibility test _____
   Legs straight _____
   Forward bending with knees bent _____
3. Hamstrings flexibility (SLR): Right _____ Left _____
4. Quadratus lumborum flexibility _____
5. Thomas Test for iliopsoas flexibility: Right _____ Left _____
6. Abdominal muscle strength _____
7. Ability to flatten lower back to floor (lying supine) _____
8. Range of shoulder motion: Right _____ Left _____
9. Length of lower extremities: Right _____ Left _____
10. Back muscle strength: Cervical erectors _____
    Erector spinae _____
    Scapulae adductors _____
11. Shoulder girdle strength:
    Abduction: Right _____ Left _____
    Adduction: Right _____ Left _____
    Flexion: Right _____ Left _____
    Extension: Right _____ Left _____
12. Static balance: Right leg _____ Left leg _____
13. Dynamic balance _____
14. Forward walking (general evaluation – broad/narrow support base, movement balance, movement flow, coordination) _____

_____
_____

X-rays, medical documents and previous diagnoses:

_____
_____

General evaluation:

_____
_____

Recommended treatment (indications/contraindications):

_____
_____

Appendix 4

Treatment report and definition of aims

Date _____

Child's name _____ Age _____

Activity duration _____ Disorder treated _____

Type of activity: Individual/Group/Integrated   (circle one)

Location of activity _____

1. Details of the problems requiring treatment (in reference to the posture and motor tests).
2. Other aspects affecting the child's condition and the treatment process (reference to family, cognitiv
    emotional and social aspects, level of motivation, cooperation, etc.)
3. Treatment aims and content matter for the coming months:

    a. _____

    b. _____

    c. _____

    d. _____

Name of therapist/instructor _____

Appendix 5

Treatment summary report

Date _____

Child's name _____ Age _____

Activity duration _____ Disorder treated _____

1. Entry condition of the child at the beginning of treatment

    _____
    _____
    _____
    _____

2. Details of treatment goals and work method selected for attaining them

    _____
    _____
    _____
    _____

3. Child's condition today (improvement/worsening of condition)

    _____
    _____
    _____
    _____

4. Recommendations for further treatment of the child

    _____
    _____
    _____
    _____

5. General comments about treating the child

    _____
    _____
    _____
    _____

Name of therapist/instructor _____

Appendix 6

Self-exercise form

Name _____ Date _____

DETAILS OF EXERCISE (DRAWING)	NUMBER OF REPETITIONS	EMPHASIS FOR PERFORMANCE
1.		
2.		
3.		
4.		
5.		
6.		
7.		
8.		
9.		
10.		
11.		
12.		
13.		
14.		
15.		
16.		
17.		
18.		
19.		
20.		

Appendix 7

Assessment of psychomotor functioning: summary table of diagnostic data

TEST AREA	1 VERY WEAK	2 WEAK	3 MODERATE	4 GOOD	5 VERY GOOD	QUALITATIVE ASSESSMENT OF MOVEMENT PATTERNS
A. BASIC SKILLS						
Crawling						
Walking						
Running						
Climbing						
Jumping on two feet						
Hopping on right foot						
Hopping on left foot						
Skipping						
Forward somersault						
B. BALL SKILLS						
Passing (throwing)						
Catching						
Bouncing						
Shooting						
Kicking a soccer ball						
Stopping a soccer ball						
Shoulder throw with a small ball						
C. FINE MOTOR SKILLS						
Buttoning						
Tying shoelaces						
Writing						
Control of fingers						
D. GENERAL MOTOR ABILITIES						
Static balance on right leg						
Static balance on left leg						
Dynamic balance						
Agility						
Speed						
General coordination						
Eye/hand coordination						
Timing						
Regulation of force						
Reaction time						
Movement flow						
Crossing midline						
General spatial orientation						

GENERAL ASSESSMENT

Assessment of psychomotor functioning: summary table of diagnostic data (*continued*)

TEST AREA	1 VERY WEAK	2 WEAK	3 MODERATE	4 GOOD	5 VERY GOOD	QUALITATIVE ASSESSMENT OF MOVEMENT PATTERNS
Personal spatial orientation						
Kinesthesis – feeling of movement						

E. BEHAVIORAL–EMOTIONAL–COGNITIVE CHARACTERISTICS

Concentration and attention						
Cooperation and motivation						
General cognitive ability						
Language and speech						
Self confidence						
Self image						
Body image						
Motor memory						
Movement planning						
Distinguishing right and left						

F. GENERAL EVALUATION

G. MAIN EMPHASES FOR TREATMENT

1.

2.

3.

4.

Index